The Complete
Acid Reflux Diet Plan

T0020757

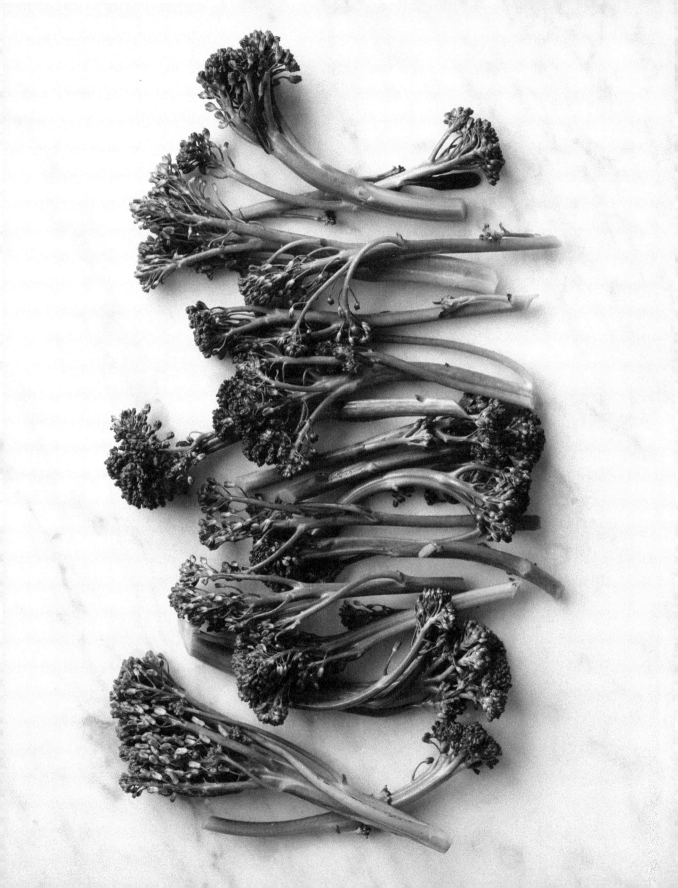

The Complete
Acid Reflux
Diet Plan

EASY MEAL PLANS and RECIPES to HEAL GERD and LPR

Nour Zibdeh, MS, RDN, CLT

ROCKRIDGE
PRESS

Copyright © 2018 by Nour Zibdeh

No part of this publication may be reproduced, stored in a retrieval system or transmitted in any form or by any means, electronic, mechanical, photocopying, recording, scanning, or otherwise, except as permitted under Sections 107 or 108 of the 1976 United States Copyright Act, without the prior written permission of the Publisher. Requests to the Publisher for permission should be addressed to the Permissions Department, Rockridge Press, 6005 Shellmound Street, Suite 175, Emeryville, CA 94608.

Limit of Liability/Disclaimer of Warranty: The Publisher and the author make no representations or warranties with respect to the accuracy or completeness of the contents of this work and specifically disclaim all warranties, including without limitation warranties of fitness for a particular purpose. No warranty may be created or extended by sales or promotional materials. The advice and strategies contained herein may not be suitable for every situation. This work is sold with the understanding that the Publisher is not engaged in rendering medical, legal, or other professional advice or services. If professional assistance is required, the services of a competent professional person should be sought. Neither the Publisher nor the author shall be liable for damages arising herefrom. The fact that an individual, organization, or website is referred to in this work as a citation and/or potential source of further information does not mean that the author or the Publisher endorses the information the individual, organization, or website may provide or recommendations they/it may make. Further, readers should be aware that websites listed in this work may have changed or disappeared between when this work was written and when it is read.

For general information on our other products and services or to obtain technical support, please contact our Customer Care Department within the United States at (866) 744-2665, or outside the United States at (510) 253-0500.

Rockridge Press publishes its books in a variety of electronic and print formats. Some content that appears in print may not be available in electronic books, and vice versa.

TRADEMARKS: Rockridge Press and the Rockridge Press logo are trademarks or registered trademarks of Callisto Media Inc. and/or its affiliates, in the United States and other countries, and may not be used without written permission. All other trademarks are the property of their respective owners. Rockridge Press is not associated with any product or vendor mentioned in this book.

Cover photography © Jennifer Davick, Anna Pustynnikova/Shutterstock

Interior photography © Jennifer Davick, ii; Cau de Sucre/Stockfood, vii; Lars Ranek/Stockfood, p.2; Stacy Grant/Stockfood, p.18; Nadine Greeff/Stocksy, p.28; Natasa Mandic/Stocksy, p.68, back cover; Nadine Greeff, p.90; Darren Muir/Stocksy, p.106; Ina Peters/ Stocksy, p.130; Jennifer Davick, p.152; Izy Hossack/Stockfood, p.170; Grafe & Unser Verlag/Stockfood, p.192; Jennifer Davick, p.210.

Author photograph © Nazia Abbas

ISBN: Print 978-1-93975-479-0 | eBook 978-1-93975-480-6

*To my parents for
always believing in me*

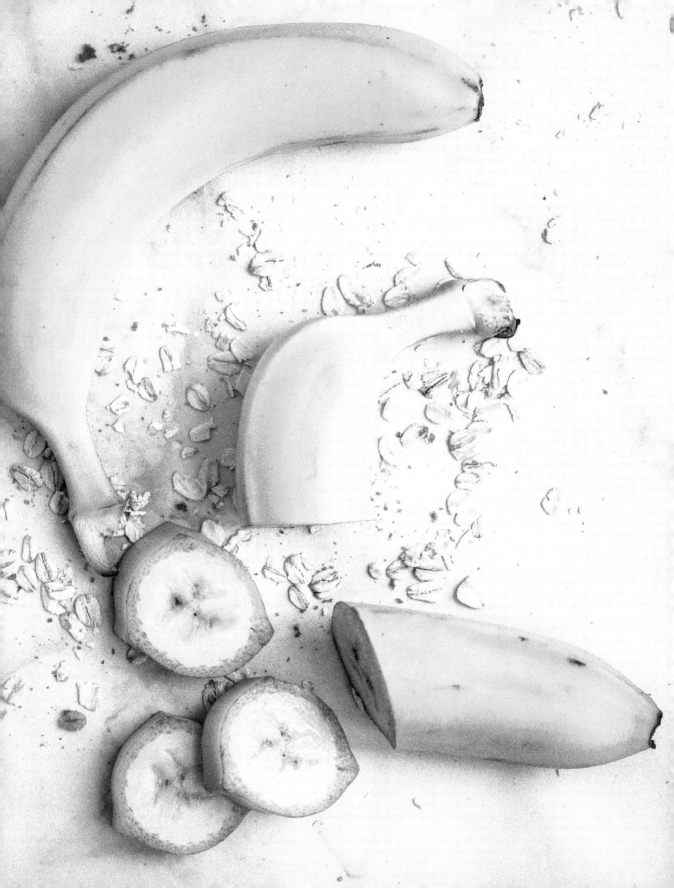

Contents

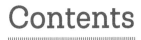

Introduction *viii*

PART I: HEALING GERD AND LPR

1 THE ROOT CAUSES OF ACID REFLUX 3

2 UNDERSTANDING THE ACID REFLUX DIET 19

3 DIFFERENT MEAL PLANS FOR DIFFERENT NEEDS 29

PART II: RECIPES THAT PREVENT ACID REFLUX

4 BREAKFAST AND BRUNCH 69

5 APPETIZERS AND SIDES 91

6 VEGETARIAN AND VEGAN 107

7 SEAFOOD AND POULTRY 131

8 BEEF AND LAMB 153

9 SNACKS AND SWEETS 171

10 SAUCES AND CONDIMENTS 193

The FDA's pH Food Lists 211

The Dirty Dozen and the Clean Fifteen™ 215

Measurements and Conversions 216

References 217   Resources 220   Recipe Index 222

Index 224

Introduction

Congratulations! You are on your way to completely eliminating your heartburn and acid reflux.

If you're like the patients who come to my practice seeking nutritional therapy for acid reflux, you're familiar with the pain and discomfort of not being able to enjoy foods you once loved. If you're one of the 50 million people who suffer from silent acid reflux, you probably feel a near-constant need to cough, have difficulty swallowing, or experience a choking sensation in your throat. Whether symptoms of heartburn or acid reflux are new to you or you've been suffering for years, I want you to know one thing: It's absolutely possible to stop the suffering, and you don't have to rely on acid-blocking medication to do it.

The great news is that you can use a food-based approach to stop acid reflux pain—and prevent it from coming back. And that's exactly what this book will help you do.

The traditional approach to acid reflux is often a prescription pad, and although acid blockers can help initially reduce the pain and the damage to the esophagus, they don't solve the root of the problem. On top of that, long-term use is associated with nutrient deficiencies and increased risk of bone fractures, among other undesirable side effects. Unfortunately, many patients go on for years taking medications that are meant to be used for a few months only.

Even when diet is considered, patients are often just given a general list of foods to avoid and then left to figure out their individual triggers on their own. Like quick-fix drug solutions, eliminating certain foods without solving the underlying trigger will keep you stuck in a lifetime of diet restriction that is neither easy nor sustainable.

According to the medical community, excess stomach acid is the main cause of heartburn and acid reflux. While this might be the case for some people, for many others the opposite is true. We produce less stomach acid as we age, yet the risk of developing acid reflux and gastroesophageal reflux disease (GERD) *increases*. So the culprit cannot be just excess stomach acid. In fact, the real problem is the presence of *any* amount of acid—small or large—in the esophagus, which is not designed to tolerate it.

My passion and training in functional nutrition made me determined to peel back the layers and uncover the underlying cause of acid hanging out in the wrong place. Acid reflux is a sign of disrupted function in the digestive tract. Most of my heartburn and acid reflux patients have other digestive complaints, too. In fact, there's an overlap between irritable bowel syndrome (IBS) and GERD.

The first time I encountered a patient with a "lump sensation" in his throat, I didn't realize it was acid reflux. He didn't complain of heartburn. He just wanted to get rid of his bloating and stomach pain. As his bloating resolved, the sensation of having a lump in his throat disappeared along with it. I've learned since then to connect the dots between the esophagus and the rest of the gut.

What makes this book different from other acid reflux books is the focus on solving the root cause, not just eliminating acidic foods. I present a complete food-based approach so you don't have to stay on a restricted diet forever. Sound good? Food is fun, a celebration, and part of who we are. You want a long-term solution so you can go back to enjoying meals without pain, and dietary changes can give you exactly that.

The Complete Acid Reflux Diet Plan includes three plans: STOP, HEAL, and REINTRODUCE. The goal of the first plan—the three-day STOP—is to get immediate relief from pain and discomfort. The second plan—the four-week HEAL—tackles the root cause of reflux to prevent stomach content from being pushed up into the esophagus. In the final plan—the four-week REINTRODUCE— you will gradually bring back some of the foods that were eliminated and learn how to tailor the plan for your own needs.

Your goal is not to eliminate acidic foods for the rest of your life. Rather, it is to be able to enjoy the foods you love and get free of those medications. When you improve digestion, heal the esophagus, restore proper function to the gut, and stop the stomach from pushing its content up, acidic foods such as berries or pineapple will not bother you anymore.

Changing your diet can be difficult and even a little overwhelming in the beginning, but the payoff will transform your life. What will you do when you no longer have pain? What activities or sports will you participate in? How will your mood and energy improve? Is the constant cough or throat clearing disrupting your work or livelihood? And how will eliminating these symptoms open opportunities you thought you could never take advantage of? What will freedom from acid reflux medications and their side effects enable you to do?

With the plans and recipes in this book, you will nourish your body and prevent serious and life-threatening damage from happening.

Food can be your medicine. Let it be.

Part One

Healing GERD and LPR

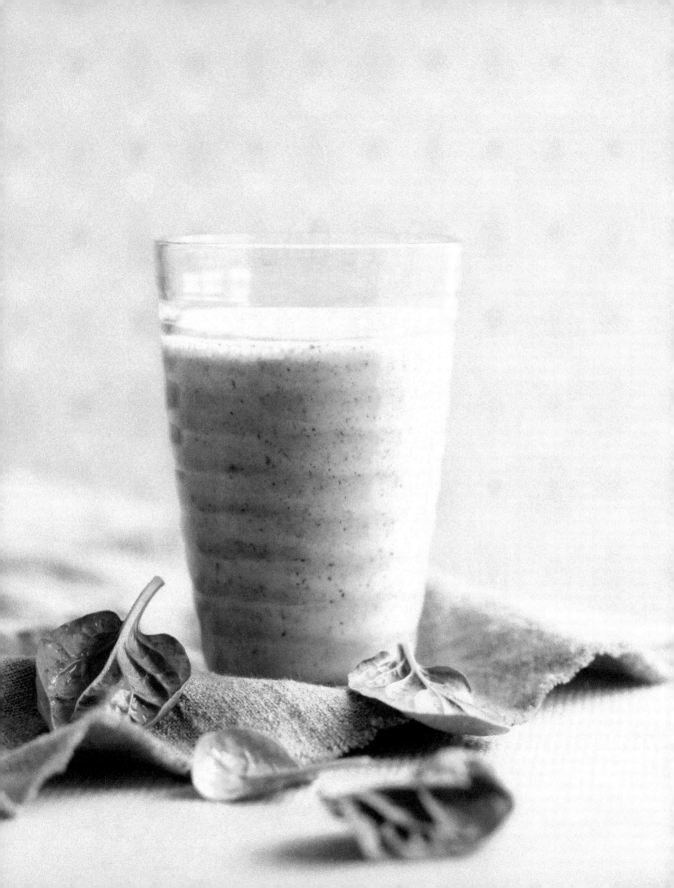

1

The Root Causes of Acid Reflux

Before diving deeply into heartburn and acid reflux, it's important to understand the basics about digestion. You'll gain a much greater appreciation for your digestive tract and the intricate balance between its components, which will empower you to make smart choices because you'll know how certain foods could cause discomfort or worsen acid reflux.

As you will discover in this chapter, acid reflux may be just the tip of the iceberg. We're going to discuss the mechanism by which reflux causes symptoms, when you should see a doctor, and how your food choices and the health of your gut interact to trigger acid reflux and heartburn.

Digestion Overview

Digestion begins in the mouth with your first bite. The smell and taste of food trigger the release of saliva, which moistens the food and helps your teeth mechanically break it down. Saliva contains the enzyme amylase, which starts the chemical digestion of amylose, the complex sugar molecule that makes up starch.

Your digestive tract is made up of muscles that move involuntarily in a sequence of contractions that resemble a wave. When you swallow, food is pushed down through the esophagus. A group of muscles called the lower esophageal sphincter (LES) separates the esophagus from the stomach and opens to allow food to enter the stomach.

The smell and taste of food also trigger the release of hydrochloric acid (HCl), often referred to as stomach acid. It creates an acidic environment that helps kill pathogens in food, changes the shape of food proteins so enzymes can tackle them better, and activates the enzyme pepsin. Pepsin is the first protein-digesting enzyme secreted by stomach cells, but it can't get to work until it is switched on by an acid. In the stomach, this acid is HCl. Once switched on, pepsin breaks large protein molecules into smaller proteins called peptides.

Pepsin and HCl work together to extract nutrients from the meals you worked hard to prepare. Pepsin unfolds protein structures so amino acids and nutrients that are bound to them can be released. For example, vitamin B_{12} needs to get released from food protein in order to attach to another protein—known as the intrinsic factor—in the stomach. Without this step, it can't be absorbed later in the small intestine. Acidity is also needed for efficient iron absorption. Studies show that long-term use of acid-blocking medications leads to iron and vitamin B_{12} malabsorption, and reducing HCl production also interferes with zinc absorption. Calcium, magnesium, copper, selenium, and niacin (vitamin B3) are other vital nutrients that may not be properly absorbed with low stomach acid. If you have heartburn, stomach pain, indigestion, bloating, or constipation after eating protein-rich foods, it's likely that pepsin is not working as properly as it should due to a low level of stomach acid.

Aside from destroying pathogens in food, acidity hinders the growth of the ulcer-producing bacteria *Helicobacter pylori* (H. pylori). Stomach acid also prevents harmful bacteria, fungus, and parasite growth in the small intestine. You can see that acidity is very much needed!

The lining of the stomach handles this harsh acidic environment by producing a thick protective mucous layer. The lining of the esophagus and throat, however, has nothing to do with stomach content, so it does not produce any protective layer. Therefore, any amount of stomach content containing pepsin and HCl that refluxes up into the esophagus will cause irritation.

Back to digestion: After a few hours of food churning and mixing in the stomach, the muscle that separates the stomach from the small intestine opens slightly. It gradually releases the stomach's contents, now a mixture of partially digested proteins, carbohydrates, and fats called chyme, into the duodenum, the first section of the small intestine. This triggers the pancreas to release bicarbonate to neutralize the acid and enzymes that aid digestion. Also, the gallbladder releases bile salts that neutralize acid, kill bacteria, aid in the breakdown and absorption of fats, and help eliminate compounds that the body no longer needs.

Food continues to move to the middle part of the small intestine, where the final steps of digestion happen. Partially digested proteins, carbohydrates, and fats are completely broken down into their single unit forms, which can then be absorbed. Vitamins and minerals are absorbed as well. The food then travels to the last part of the small intestine, where water, more vitamins, and bile salts are absorbed. What is left of your food at this point is undigested material and fiber that pass to the large intestine.

In the large intestine, or colon, more water and electrolytes are absorbed. The colon also hosts trillions of organisms that represent 500 different species, collectively known as your gut flora. There, beneficial bacteria ferment undigested fiber and produce short-chain fatty acids that directly nourish the cells of your intestine. They also help us extract more nutrients from food, produce some vitamins (such as vitamin K_2), and fight harmful bacteria.

The muscle contractions of the digestive tract continue to push food remnants through the colon. By this point, it's mostly waste and exits the body in the form of stool. It usually takes from 33 to 47 hours after you eat for what is remaining of your meal to pass.

More Than Just Heartburn

While heartburn is the most common symptom of acid reflux, it's just the tip of the iceberg. In fact, when I talk about acid reflux, I often just use the word *reflux*, because acid is not the problem—it just gets the bad rap. *Reflux* is the problem. To heal heartburn and silent reflux symptoms, you must uncover the causes of reflux and address them.

When reflux happens on a weekly basis, you will be diagnosed with GERD. Long-term reflux can change the shape of the cells that line the lower part of the esophagus. This condition is known as Barrett's esophagus, and it's associated with increased risk for esophageal cancer. That's why it's important to take action if you have reflux.

Some people have acid reflux without the classic heartburn symptoms. Laryngopharyngeal reflux (LPR), also referred to as silent acid reflux, can be more serious because people don't connect symptoms in the throat to a problem in the stomach. Fifty million Americans don't know that they have silent acid reflux! They may experience frequent coughing, postnasal drip, hoarseness in the voice, difficulty swallowing, a lump sensation in the throat, choking episodes, and even asthma! The damage can be happening for years, even decades, before they realize it or do something about it.

Fortunately, you have picked up this book, so you now have the tools to eliminate your symptoms and reduce your risk of serious long-term damage.

When people experience heartburn, they typically just zero in on stomach acid. Most health care attempts to heal acid reflux involve a prescription for an acid-blocking medication. In 2014, 13 million prescriptions for Nexium, a proton pump inhibitor (PPI), were written—making it the second most sold drug in the United States, with sales of $1.5 million. Pharmaceutical companies want you to believe that too much stomach acid causes acid reflux because that's good for their bottom lines. But acid-blocking medications are not the right solution for everyone. Ten percent of people taking PPIs report no improvement in symptoms, and 15 to 20 percent experience side effects such as gas, bloating, nausea, diarrhea, and abdominal pain.

Reflux, the presence of stomach content in the esophagus, is a sign that something in the digestive tract has gone awry. A retrospective study on more than 6,000 patients found that 64 percent of people with IBS also had GERD, and 34 percent of people with GERD had IBS. The authors of this study, published in the *World Journal of Gastroenterology* in March 2010, attributed the overlap between the two conditions to a common dysfunction in the digestive tract. In other words, something else might be causing both GERD and IBS. Reflux is just a sign that something in your gut is wrong. To solve the problem once and for all, we must look beyond stomach acid.

In the book *Dropping Acid: The Reflux Diet Cookbook and Cure*, Drs. Jamie Koufman and Jordan Stern describe pepsin molecules—the enzyme that digests protein—as lobsters with big, aggressive claws. The lobster claws attach to the cells of the esophagus for the first time when the content of the stomach splashes up. They hang in there long after the initial splash and start eating tissue whenever acid is present. The minute you swallow an acidic food, whether it's a healthy strawberry or a can of soda, the lobsters get active, eating away at your tissue and causing symptoms. Acidic foods that were harmless now become major offenders. Every time you reflux, more lobsters climb into your esophagus.

The question is, why is the stomach content refluxing upward? Shouldn't it move down toward the rest of the digestive tract? In a normal, healthy situation, the LES muscles stay shut, the stomach properly completes its digestive steps, and then the pyloric valve gradually opens and releases chyme into the duodenum. But when you have reflux, the food moves in the wrong direction.

The underlying cause of reflux is increased pressure from the abdomen, known as intra-abdominal pressure (IAP), which pushes the contents of the

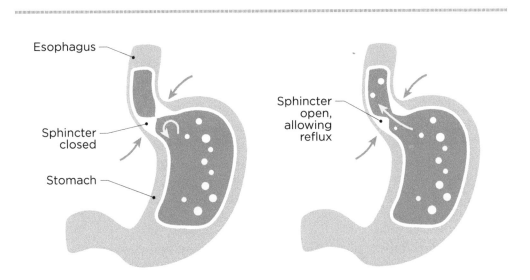

This figure shows the content of the stomach, including pepsin and HCl, refluxing upward in response to increased pressure from the stomach and abdomen and weakened LES muscles. In people with GERD (left), stomach content backs up into the esophagus, causing heartburn and esophagitis (inflammation in the esophagus). In people with LPR, the stomach content reaches the larynx and throat (right), and they may experience hoarseness, difficulty swallowing, chronic coughing, and other symptoms.

stomach up. Slow and disrupted digestion, excessive fermentation, loosened LES muscles, and fat accumulation in the abdomen contribute to IAP and reflux. We will explore each one of those in more detail.

The spread of commercially packaged acidified foods adds insult to injury. In the 1970s, Title 21 of the U.S. Food and Drug Administration's Code of Federal Regulations allowed manufacturers to use acids to create more shelf-stable foods. Remember that acid kills bacteria! These preserved foods can maintain a pH value of less than 4.6, preventing the growth of *Clostridium botulinum* bacteria, which produces a potent toxin capable of causing a lethal disease called botulism.

Acidified foods include commercial sauces, condiments, pickles, marinades, salad dressings, liquid energy shots, nutrition shakes, and many more. If the ingredients list contains vinegar (acetic acid) or citric, lactic, malic, or phosphoric acid, the food is acidic. Americans have come to depend more on these convenient acidic foods, and in combination with imbalances in the digestive tract, it's no wonder that more people of all ages are experiencing heartburn and acid reflux.

Common Symptoms and Conditions

People experience the classic symptoms of heartburn soon after eating. Large meals that are greasy, starchy, or spicy are more problematic. Symptoms are worse if they eat too quickly, or lie down or exercise soon after eating. With silent reflux (LPR), the symptoms can be chronic or intermittent. They may happen around meals or away from meals, during the day or at night.

These are the most common symptoms of reflux, GERD, and LPR:

- Heartburn
- Regurgitation
- Chest pain
- Shortness of breath
- Hoarseness
- Difficulty swallowing
- "Lump" feeling in the throat
- Choking sensation
- Chronic cough
- Chronic throat clearing
- Postnasal drip
- Difficulty breathing
- Intermittent airway obstruction
- Wheezing

The Reflux Symptom Index (RSI) below is a screening tool, developed by Drs. Jamie Koufman and Jordan Stern, that can help you determine if you have

LPR. It doesn't replace a complete medical assessment and diagnosis, but it allows you to see how many related symptoms you have and how severe your symptoms are. A score of 15 or higher is an indicator of LPR, but even if you have a lower value and suspect that you have it, it's not a bad idea to check with an ENT (ear, nose, and throat) specialist.

Within the last month, how did the following problem affect you? (0–5 rating scale, where 0 = no problem and 5 = severe problem)

Hoarseness or problem with your voice	0	1	2	3	4	5
Clearing your throat	0	1	2	3	4	5
Excess throat mucus or postnasal drip	0	1	2	3	4	5
Difficulty swallowing foods, liquids, or pills	0	1	2	3	4	5
Cough after you ate or after lying down	0	1	2	3	4	5
Breathing difficulties or choking episodes	0	1	2	3	4	5
Troublesome or annoying cough	0	1	2	3	4	5
Sensation of something sticking in your throat	0	1	2	3	4	5
Heartburn, chest pain, indigestion, or stomach acid coming up	0	1	2	3	4	5

Total

From Dropping Acid: The Reflux Diet Cookbook and Cure, reprinted by permission of Drs. Jamie Koufman and Jordan Stern.

When Should I See a Doctor?

If you've tried my eating plans and modified your diet for two to four weeks and still continue to experience symptoms, you may want to see a gastroenterologist or ENT doctor to see if there's anything more serious going on. They'll be able to screen you for various disorders ranging from Barrett's esophagus to ulcers and cancer. If there's a serious condition, the sooner you discover it, the better your chances of making a full recovery.

EMERGENCY TIPS TO TREAT FLARE-UPS

If you have heartburn flare-up, you can try one of these remedies:

- **Ginger.** To boost digestion, make a ginger tea by mixing 1 teaspoon of grated fresh ginger in 1 cup of warm water. You may add ½ teaspoon of pure maple syrup if desired.

- **Aloe vera plant.** You may have seen aloe vera drinks in stores, but these tend to contain sugars and preservatives. Instead, keep an aloe leaf in your refrigerator or grow a plant in your home. Cut a piece of aloe, peel the green hard skin, and you'll be left with the clear, gooey part. Mix it into a smoothie to take advantage of its many digestive benefits.

- **Bone broth.** Sipping warm bone broth can help soothe the lining of your throat and esophagus.

- **Get up!** Or if you're lying down, elevate your head with pillows so your head is higher than your torso.

- **Rest.** If you're running around catching up on work or errands, stop and take a moment to calm down. Sit down for five minutes and take deep breaths.

- **Walk it off.** If you overate, go out for a light walk. Avoid jumping or any exercise that involves too much shaking.

If you have any of these symptoms, you may want to schedule an appointment with a specialist sooner rather than later:

- Severe heartburn that happens more than twice a week despite following the plans in this book and/or taking over-the-counter acid-suppressing medications for more than two weeks
- Severe chest pain right after eating that almost feels like a heart attack (This usually calls for a trip to your gastroenterologist, but of course chest pain may also mean a heart attack. If it's accompanied by other heart attack signs such as pain and tightness in the neck and arms, light-headedness, abnormal heartbeat, or anxiety, call 911 right away.)

- Extreme coughing that wakes you up at night, especially if it's so severe that you feel you will suffocate or run out of breath
- A cough that lasts more than three months despite normal chest X-rays and ruling out any chest or throat infections
- Pain or difficulty when swallowing, a choking sensation, or a constant feeling of a lump in the throat
- Hoarseness in the morning that gets worse during the day, or a scratchy voice
- A feeling of narrowing or obstruction in the esophagus
- Nausea or vomiting, especially if vomiting blood, as it can be a sign of esophageal ulcer
- Blood in the stool or black bowel movements

To help your doctor make a diagnosis, keep a record of your symptoms, the times they happen, and their severity. Record when, what, and how much you eat. Tracking your stress level and sleep will reveal how your environment affects your symptoms. Follow the STOP and HEAL plans in chapter 3 until your scheduled doctor's appointment. Your symptoms will likely improve, but if they don't, your doctor will want to know that.

Medical tests and doctors' visits may seem unpleasant or stressful. However, ruling out more serious medical conditions will alleviate anxiety and allow you to focus on preparing and eating the right foods. And if the tests do come back with bad news, you'll be able to start treatment sooner and have a better outcome.

The Connection between the Gut, Diet, and Acid Reflux

As I emphasized before, all parts of the digestive tract must work harmoniously, or else symptoms, including reflux and heartburn, can start to occur. In this section, we'll talk about disruptions in gut function, food choices, medications, and certain health conditions that can lead to reflux. It doesn't mean that you have these conditions or that you need to stop a medication. Talk with your health care provider, inquire about testing, and come up with a plan for tapering off medications if possible.

When digestion is slow, food sits in the stomach for too long and is more likely to reflux upward. Fatty and greasy meals slow down gastric emptying—how quickly the stomach releases its content to the duodenum.

What slows down digestion? One cause is a low stomach acid level. This may be surprising, as you're used to hearing that too much acid causes reflux! Remember that acid is necessary to activate pepsin and initiate protein digestion. Long-term use of acid-blocking medications is shown to reduce HCl production.

We produce less HCl as we age. A study in the *Journal of the American Geriatrics Society* found that 30 percent of men and women over the age of 60 have atrophic gastritis, a condition where there is diminished HCl production, as well as anemia and vitamin B_{12} deficiency. Another study in the same journal found that 27 percent of the 3,484 participants had diminished HCl, and the percentage was highest among women between the ages of 80 and 89. A third study, in the journal *Gastroenterology*, found that 40 percent of menopausal women had no signs of HCl production.

A 2016 review in *Rama University Journal of Medical Sciences* lists aging, acid-blocking medications (antacids, PPIs, and H1/H2 blockers), *H. pylori* infection, gastric bypass surgery, chicken pox, and intestinal dysbiosis (imbalance in gut microbes) as causes of low stomach acid. Symptoms of low gastric acid include bloating, diarrhea, constipation, heartburn, indigestion, hair loss in women, malaise, food allergies, among others, based on a literature review in *Alternative Medicine Review*. It also links low stomach acid to gut dysbiosis, chronic yeast or parasite infections, iron deficiency, adult acne, undigested food in the stool, and weak or cracked fingernails.

Fifty percent of the population is estimated to have the common stomach bacteria *H. pylori*. The first infection can happen only if stomach acidity is reduced, such as when taking acid-blocking medications. Once in the stomach, the bacteria further reduce HCl production to favor their own survival. If you have heartburn, acid reflux, or LPR, ask your doctor to test you for *H. pylori*.

Since low stomach acid can contribute to reflux, you might wonder if you should in fact eat acidic foods to help compensate for low acidity in the stomach. The problem with eating acidic foods before healing completely is that they will activate pepsin in the throat and esophagus and cause pain and irritation. Remember that a thick mucous layer protects the stomach, but that is not the case in any other part of the digestive tract, leaving those other parts vulnerable to damage from acid.

Some medical conditions can slow down digestion. Underactive thyroid, or hypothyroidism, slows down peristalsis, the muscle motion that moves food through the digestive tract. Gastroparesis is a condition marked by the stomach taking too long to empty. Nerve damage in people with uncontrolled diabetes, and disruptions in nerve signals as in Parkinson's disease, can also slow down digestion, as can tricyclic antidepressants, such as amitriptyline. Share your concerns with your doctor and ask that these conditions be screened for and ruled out.

EXCESSIVE FERMENTATION

Excessive fermentation combined with slow digestion and low HCl is triple trouble. The bacteria in your small intestine love sugars and other carbohydrates! They eat them up through fermentation and produce gases that push the stomach content up to the esophagus. While all carbohydrates are easy and delicious food for bacteria, a set of carbohydrates known as FODMAPs tend to cause the most fermentation. We will talk more about foods that contain FODMAPs in chapter 2.

You may wonder what your small intestine has to do with reflux. Consider this: If just 30 grams of carbohydrates escape digestion, bacterial fermentation produces 10 liters of gas! Imagine almost three gallons of gas in your gut! That's enough to increase intra-abdominal pressure and contribute to reflux.

Traditional anti-reflux diets focus on reducing fats and completely ignore the effect of carbohydrate fermentation. A noteworthy study in *Digestive Diseases and Sciences* showed that a low-carbohydrate diet improved GERD symptoms to a degree similar to the effect of PPI medications. Many of my patients who follow a low-carbohydrate diet confirm this and report improvement in heartburn and other digestive symptoms. This means you can manage GERD with diet and lifestyle without depending on medications. Since we're committed to getting to the root of the problem to restore function to all—not just one part—of your digestive system, removing fermentable carbohydrates will be an important part of your HEAL plan.

This is a good time to point out a condition known as small intestinal bacterial overgrowth (SIBO). If you recall our discussion of the gut, most bacteria reside in the large, not the small, intestine. Stomach acid inhibits bacterial overgrowth in the small intestine. In SIBO, bacteria migrate to the small intestine, where they have access to carbohydrates before you can digest and absorb them. The result of carbohydrate fermentation is gas production that causes bloating, flatulence, stomach pain, diarrhea, or constipation. If you have these along with heartburn, and removing FODMAP foods in the HEAL plan significantly improves your symptoms, you may have SIBO.

Acid-suppressing medications are associated with SIBO which, in return, worsens acid reflux. A 2000 study published in the *Journal of Gastrointestinal Surgery* showed that 11 of 30 people with GERD who took a PPI for at least three months developed SIBO. In contrast, only 1 of 10 people with GERD who were off medications developed SIBO. Two additional studies found that treating SIBO with antibiotics improved GERD symptoms and helped strengthen LES muscles.

SIBO causes pain, discomfort, gut inflammation, nutrient deficiencies, and fatigue. It can be one of the root causes of GERD. Ask your doctor to properly test you.

WEAKENED LES MUSCLES

With age, the LES muscles that separate the esophagus from the stomach can weaken and allow stomach content to reflux upward. Combine that with increased IAP from fermentable carbohydrates, fatty foods, slow digestion, low stomach acid, and bacterial growth, and you have the perfect storm for reflux, GERD, and LPR.

Some foods have been associated with weakening the LES muscles. These include caffeinated foods and drinks such as coffee, tea, chocolate, and energy drinks, as well as peppermint and bell peppers. Smoking and alcohol consumption also weaken the LES muscles. Carbonated beverages, even the no-calorie versions, increase IAP, which eventually affects the tone of LES muscles.

Some medications can also weaken the LES muscles. These include calcium channel blockers (blood pressure medications), bisphosphonates (osteoporosis medications), sedatives, and sleeping pills. If you're taking one of those, discuss alternatives with your doctor.

ABDOMINAL OBESITY

Addressing overweight and obesity is beyond the scope of this book. However, accumulating weight around the belly increases IAP, which contributes to heartburn and acid reflux.

FOOD SENSITIVITIES

If you continue to have symptoms despite an anti-inflammatory diet and the plans outlined in this book, it's possible that you have developed food sensitivities. Food sensitivities happen when your immune cells can't recognize foods as "safe" and start to react to them. Symptoms include heartburn, bloating, stomach pain, diarrhea, constipation, headaches, migraines, skin issues, muscle and joint pain, brain fog, and fatigue.

Food sensitivities are common, affecting from 30 to 40 percent of the population. The foods that you may be reacting to are very individual to you and your immune system. You may react to healthy foods such as kale, almonds, or avocado! You may also develop sensitivities to natural or synthetic food chemicals.

Food sensitivities are not the same as food allergies, so you may have food sensitivities despite normal results from food allergy tests. Symptoms of food sensitivities are neither acute nor immediate. It may take up to 72 hours after eating for symptoms to surface. Since you may eat dozens of different foods and food chemicals in this timeframe, it becomes complicated to uncover the problem foods just with a food diary.

Someone may live with food sensitivities for years before they realize that their immune system is off. While certain foods such as gluten, dairy, soy, corn, eggs, fish, and shellfish are commonly recognized as allergenic, I find that the best way to truly address food sensitivities is through testing and an individualized plan. If you suspect this is your issue, you can read more about food sensitivity testing on my website at NourZibdeh.com/MRT.

Solving the obesity and overweight epidemic is by no means an easy or straightforward equation. If that were the case, we wouldn't be seeing obesity rates skyrocket! While consuming large amounts of food—more than the body can burn through daily activity and exercise—contributes to obesity, there's more to it than that.

Inflammation is a major contributor to obesity. Inflammatory foods—those containing too much sugar, fats, processed and damaged oils, and preservatives—contribute to accumulating weight and fat around the belly. Commercially preserved foods are also acidic, making heartburn, GERD, and LPR symptoms worse. When people consume a diet high in processed foods, they often fail to eat nutritious, antioxidant-packed foods that help fight inflammation.

Stress can also make you accumulate weight around the belly. It has a physiological effect as it makes you produce more cortisol (stress hormone) and insulin (fat storage hormone). When you're stressed out, you eat mindlessly. You eat too quickly, you don't chew your food thoroughly enough, and you don't savor your meals, leaving you still hungry for more. Your brain and your gut are intimately connected through the nervous system. Anxiety, or feeling like you're in a fight-or-flight situation, will disrupt or shut down digestion and cause heartburn and stomach pain.

Most people think of responsibilities, finances, chores, deadlines, significant others, kids, and social interaction when discussing stress. But stress can be internal, too. Lack of sleep, nutrient deficiencies, inflammatory foods, and irritation in any organ (including the throat and esophagus) are all sources of stress. Having SIBO, *H. pylori*, or any other chronic infection will keep your body in a state of stress and inflammation. If you want to reduce your abdominal obesity to help with acid reflux and heartburn, look at your mind and body from a holistic perspective.

Lifestyle Solutions for Acid Reflux

When it comes to health, your story doesn't end with your genes. You write your own story with the lifestyle choices you make.

When, what, and how much you eat all affect reflux symptoms. How you move your body and manage stress are also very important. If you follow the plans in this book without also making the right lifestyle choices, you will be trying to push a large boulder uphill.

Help your body heal from heartburn, acid reflux, GERD, and LPR with these lifestyle solutions:

Wear loose clothing. Tight clothes can push on your stomach and increase IAP.

Wait three hours after dinner before lying down to sleep. Elevate your pillow or incline your bed when you sleep to reduce the effect of gravity on reflux.

Avoid late-night snacks. This will help you lose weight, too.

Avoid drinking with your meals. Fluids dilute stomach acid and reduce the capacity of digestive activity. The result is indigestion, slowed gastric emptying, more fermentation, and more reflux. Drink water 30 minutes before or an hour after your meals.

Avoid all carbonated beverages. They increase IAP and reflux.

Eat in a relaxed environment. Don't eat when upset or emotional. Avoid heated conversations during meals.

Slow down and sit down to eat. Most people are constantly on the go and don't allow themselves time to eat. Take a few minutes to do a deep breathing exercise to slow down and transition to your meal. Give yourself at least 20 minutes to eat.

Remove distractions during mealtimes. Turn off the TV, phones, and social media when eating. Focus on the food and make it a mindful experience.

If you smoke, quit. It causes inflammation in too many parts of your body.

Avoid alcohol. It can irritate the throat, esophagus, and stomach. It may also weaken the LES muscles.

Manage your stress. I've given up on telling people to eliminate stress. Stress is inevitable. We can't control our environment, but we can control how we react to it. Find ways to eliminate or reduce negative and sabotaging thoughts, and replace them with positive and empowering ones. Don't make assumptions about people or things. Don't let uncertainty or fear of the future debilitate you. Practice positive habits so you are confident and grounded no matter what life throws at you.

Meditate. Give yourself five minutes in the morning, before your meals, or between chores or activities to slow down. Close your eyes and take deep breaths. Meditation has many health benefits for the mind and the body, especially your gut, thanks to the brain-gut connection. If you don't know how to meditate, there are lots of online videos or apps to help you get started.

If you have sleep apnea, wear your device. Chronic snoring, congestion, fatigue, and daytime sleepiness are signs of sleep apnea. You are at an increased risk if you are overweight. Talk to your doctor if you suspect that you have sleep apnea, so you can get proper testing and diagnosis.

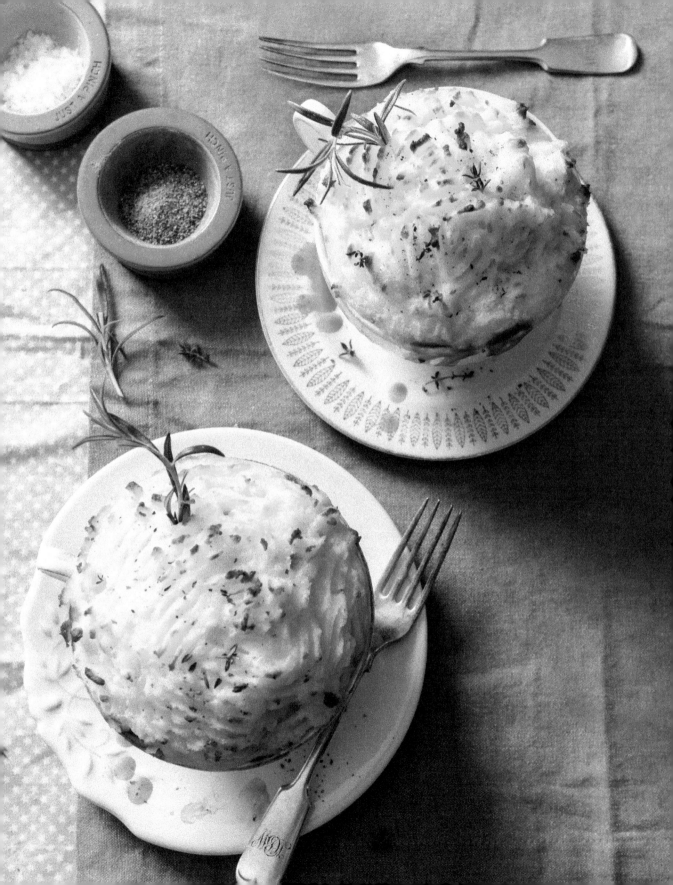

2

Understanding the Acid Reflux Diet

In this chapter, we are going to discuss the different aspects of the diet to heal acid reflux, heartburn, GERD, and LPR. Remember that my goal isn't to just give you a list of acidic foods to avoid. I want you to follow a plan that will solve the underlying cause of reflux so you can enjoy berries, pineapples, tomatoes, and citrus again! And if your heartburn, GERD, or LPR comes with other digestive issues, you will notice a major overall improvement in how you feel.

A Healthy Diet to Treat GERD and LPR

When embarking on a therapeutic diet, people often focus on what they can't have. Instead, as you read through this chapter and the next, remember that there are still lots of foods to enjoy. Just skim through the recipes to see for yourself! You might miss some of your favorites, but keep in mind that you're not going to eat this way for the rest of your life.

In a short period of time, you will get rid of your symptoms, heal your digestive tract, and restore proper digestion. When you do that, those foods that used to trigger pain and discomfort will no longer bother you. If, however, symptoms persist, you will have a better understanding of some of the imbalances that may happen in the gut, and be better equipped to discuss your health concerns with your doctor.

In the next few weeks, you will be eating these types of food:

Low-acid. In the first two plans, you will choose vegetables, fruit, fats, proteins, carbohydrates, spices, and seasonings that are low in acid. In the third plan, you will start reintroducing some acidic foods to see if you can tolerate them. Of course, these will be nutrient-rich whole foods such as berries, not soda or processed acidic foods.

Low-FODMAP. In addition to low-acid foods, you will eat foods low in FODMAPs during the HEAL plan. Don't worry about the term just yet—I'll explain it in a bit. The recipes in the second section of the book contain only low-FODMAPs foods, so I've done the work for you.

Anti-inflammatory. You will eat healthy essential fats such as salmon, nuts, and olive oil; healthy lean proteins; herbs such as thyme, rosemary, and oregano; vegetables such as kale and spinach; and other known anti-inflammatory agents such as ginger, turmeric, and aloe vera. In the third plan, when it's time to bring back some of the foods you eliminated, you're going to stick to an anti-inflammatory way of eating. Trust me, you will love how your body feels and won't want to eat sugary, greasy, and processed foods as often again!

High-fiber. Fiber helps you have regular bowel movements, sweeping out waste and toxins that build up in the gut. It can reduce the risk of colon cancer, and lower cholesterol and blood sugar levels. While fiber reduces the amount of cholesterol and glucose you absorb from food, research is now showing that high-fiber foods prevent or reverse these conditions because fiber supports healthy bacteria balance. In fact, a study published in the journal Circulation Research identified 34 types of beneficial bacteria that improve good cholesterol (HDL) levels, while another study linked imbalanced gut flora to increased level of the bad cholesterol (LDL).

All three plans in this book eliminate greasy and sugary foods and those made with processed and artificial ingredients. If a product contains an ingredient you can't spell or recognize, put it back on the shelf. You want to eat foods made by nature, not in a factory!

In the STOP plan, you will eliminate acidic foods and common reflux triggers such as coffee, tea, mint, chocolate, and pepper. In the HEAL plan, you will remove foods that increase fermentation and IAP, both of which worsen reflux. This step is necessary to eventually be able to tolerate some acidic vegetables and fruits and taper the use of medications. After four weeks, you will start the REINTRODUCE plan, where you methodically add foods back to help you identify your own personal triggers. Hopefully, you won't have too many triggers and you'll able to eat the most flexible and varied diet without pain, discomfort, or long-term side effects.

Acidic Foods Overview

Since acidic foods and acidity frequently come up, it's a good idea to go over the pH scale so you have a full understanding of the discussion. A pH of 7 is considered neutral. Anything lower than that is acidic, and anything higher is alkaline, or basic.

Pepsin, the stomach enzyme, is activated in acidic environments. It's at 100 percent activity at a pH of 2 and continues to be very active at a pH of 5. In case you're wondering, cola hovers at 2.8! If you have pepsin in your esophagus as you chug down soda, those lobster claws will eat up the sensitive lining, causing pain, irritation, and scarring.

Pepsin activity drops to only 10 percent at a pH of 6 and it's finally inactive at 7. Most vegetables, legumes, dairy, and protein have a pH of 7. It is, however, impossible to sustain a balanced diet that contains only foods with a pH of 7 or higher to guarantee no pepsin activity, which is why it's important to heal the underlying causes of reflux so you don't have pepsin in the wrong part of your gut. Remember that pepsin activation and acidity are very important in the stomach, just not in the throat or esophagus.

You can find a full list of foods and their pH values on page 211.

WHAT'S THE DEAL WITH ALKALINE OR PH-BALANCING DIETS?

Alkaline or pH-balancing diets can be a little confusing when discussing heartburn, GERD, and LPR. There's a difference between the acidity of a food as you eat it and the residue (sometimes called "ash") it leaves behind after its digestion, absorption, and metabolism. Foods can leave either an alkaline or an acidic residue.

Alkaline diets—those that leave an alkaline residue—are thought to improve health by balancing the acidic residue produced by some foods. The claim is that acid leads to cancers, osteoporosis, and other unfavorable conditions. Green leafy vegetables, lemon juice, raw apple cider vinegar, among other foods, leave an alkaline residue, while animal proteins and beans leave an acidic residue. People who use these diets measure the pH of their urine to track their body's acidity.

Explaining alkaline diets, their pros and cons, research, and biochemistry is beyond the scope of this book. If an alkaline diet makes you feel better, it's possibly because you end up eating a lot more vegetables than you used to, which are packed with antioxidants, fiber, vitamins, and minerals. You also remove processed foods, processed fats, and excess sugar on alkaline diets, and we all know how your body feels when you nix those.

In this book, we are eliminating foods that have an acidic pH, not foods that leave an acid residue. These are very different things! Any food with a pH value of 5 or less that passes through your throat and esophagus will activate pepsin and cause symptoms. That's why we're removing lemon juice, apple cider vinegar, berries, and other fruit. Despite leaving an alkaline "ash," they will irritate your esophagus. Once you address the underlying cause and heal your throat and esophagus, there will no longer be pepsin to worry about! You will then be able to enjoy foods that leave an alkaline residue such as lemon juice and raw apple cider vinegar.

The acronym FODMAP stands for **F**ermentable **o**ligosaccharides (multiple sugars), **d**isaccharides (double sugars), **m**onosaccharides (single sugars), **A**nd **P**olyols (sugar alcohols). Don't stress too much about these terms! All you need to know is that they are types of carbohydrates that are easily fermented in the gut by bacteria.

You might wonder what the intestines have to do with acid reflux between the stomach and esophagus. But remember that a mere 30 grams of carbohydrates in the gut can produce 10 liters of gases—about three gallons—if they escape digestion. The gases will increase IAP and lead to reflux. You are more likely to react to FODMAP foods if you have SIBO, *H. pylori*, or gut dysbiosis.

When considering the effect of FODMAPs, think of your body as a bucket. As you eat more and more FODMAPs, your bucket will eventually reach a threshold

HIGH-FODMAP FOODS

TYPE OF FODMAPS	FOODS
Lactose	Buttermilk, ice cream, kefir, milk, soft cheeses, yogurt
Fructose	Apples, agave, fruit juices, high fructose corn syrup, honey, mango, nectarine, peaches, pears, watermelon
Fructan	Artichoke, barley, beets, celery, dates, garlic, grapefruit, leek, onion, rye, shallot, tomato paste and sauce, watermelon, wheat
Galactans	Beans, lentils, peas, soy
Polyols	Apples, apricots, avocado, cauliflower, mushrooms, nectarines, peaches, pears, sweet potato, sweeteners that end with -*ol* such as sorbitol, mannitol, etc.

WHAT ABOUT PREBIOTICS?

Prebiotics are a type of fiber that feed your gut flora and promote the activity of beneficial bacteria, leading to improved health and well-being for you. Despite their health benefits, if you have gut dysbiosis or SIBO, prebiotics may exacerbate symptoms like stomach pain, gas, bloating, heartburn, diarrhea, or constipation.

Foods high in prebiotics include asparagus, under-ripe bananas, chicory root, garlic, sunchokes, dandelion, green leek, onions, and whole wheat. They also show up in probiotic supplements as FOS or inulin in the ingredients list.

A low-FODMAP diet is low in prebiotics. While this will give you immediate short-term relief, this diet is not meant to be followed long-term. Prebiotics are necessary for nourishing your intestinal cells and maintaining a healthy gut flora. You need to investigate why you can't tolerate these healthy fibers and fix the underlying cause. Afterward, you'll be able to enjoy them again and get their health benefits. Discuss this issue with your health care provider, as the root causes are different from one person to another.

and overflow. That overflow point varies from one person to another. Some of my patients can introduce a small amount of FODMAPs here and there without a problem, while others can't tolerate even a tiny bit. Because you can't predict how much and how quickly your body will ferment a high-FODMAPs food, it's better to eliminate them completely during the HEAL plan.

You will notice in the next chapter that some grains and starches are low in FODMAPs and allowed in your plan. These include rice, quinoa, gluten-free oats, buckwheat, amaranth, millet, and white potato. While they are low in fermentable carbohydrates, they still contain starches and other carbohydrates, bacteria's favorite foods! Some people can't tolerate any starches or grains, including the low-FODMAP ones. If your reflux is accompanied by severe stomach pain, gas, bloating, diarrhea, or constipation, or if you've been told that you have IBS, and you still have symptoms despite following the HEAL plan, cut out all grains and see if your reflux and heartburn improve.

Dietary Rules for the Acid Reflux Diet

To get the best possible results, follow these guidelines as you plan for your meals and snacks:

Eat slowly and chew your food thoroughly. Mechanical digestion happens in the mouth. If you don't chew your food properly, your stomach will need to work harder to break it down. Food will sit longer in the stomach, and the stomach content is more likely to push up into the esophagus. Aim for chewing each bite at least 15 times.

Avoid fried and greasy foods. You can use some olive oil or avocado oil to sauté meals. You can have up to 2 tablespoons of allowed nuts (see the food tables in chapter 3) at a time as a snack or a garnish. You can even have a slice or stick of cheese for a snack. But meals that are loaded with cheese or oils, typically from fried and greasy foods or a large amount of butter, will sit longer in the stomach and cause reflux.

Avoid processed and prepackaged foods and drinks, especially those with added dietary acid. If the ingredients list contains acetic acid (vinegar) or citric, lactic, malic, or phosphoric acid, the food is too acidic.

Avoid artificial sweeteners. Sucralose, found in Splenda, has been found to affect the acidity of the gut, disrupting the natural balance between good and bad bacteria and yeast. Long-term studies on all artificial sweeteners find that people who heavily use them still gain weight around the belly. You're not doing your body a favor by choosing diet soda! You're better off not drinking soda at all.

Eat smaller meals. The right meal size is unique to each individual. Start by using a salad plate or by eating half or two-thirds of your current meal size. Each meal should keep you feeling satisfied for about three hours.

Don't graze during the day. While it's important to not eat large portions, the solution is not to eat all the time. Your digestive tract goes through a cleaning motion that pushes down waste and by-products to exit in the stool and keeps bacteria from migrating to the small intestine. This cleaning motion needs two to three hours to complete, and it gets disrupted every time you eat. In people with slow digestive motility, it may take up to four hours. Time your meals to be at least three hours apart, and give your digestive tract at least 12 hours at night to reset, repair, and clean up.

Eat a lighter meal at dinner. If you tend to come home late from work, have your main meal at lunch and eat a healthy snack for dinner.

Choose low-acid foods during the STOP and HEAL plans. These are foods with a pH value of 6 or higher. Most pepsin activity is at a pH of 5 or less, and foods with lower pH will irritate your esophagus until your stomach stops refluxing. Page 211 lists the pH values of foods, and chapter 3 includes tables of foods to enjoy and others to eliminate.

Remove foods that irritate the throat or esophagus or weaken the LES muscles during the STOP and HEAL plans. These include caffeine, chocolate, tea, coffee, mint, and bell pepper.

Remove acidic foods, common reflux triggers, and foods high in FODMAPs during the HEAL plan. Use the tables in chapter 3 for easier navigation.

Maintain a low-acid and low-FODMAP diet and reintroduce foods one at a time during the REINTRODUCE plan. I will give you instructions and more details on this in chapter 3. Remember that you will prioritize healthy anti-inflammatory foods, such as berries and avocado, before others.

What about Beverages and Drinks?

Beverages can be a problem for GERD and LPR because they cause indigestion. When you take in too much fluid with your meals, digestive enzymes in the stomach, including pepsin and HCl, get diluted. It becomes more difficult for food to be digested and more likely that food will remain longer in the stomach, causing more reflux. That's why I recommend drinking water 30 minutes before or at least an hour after your meals. If you must take a medication or supplement with your food, drink just enough to swallow the pills.

Sweetened and carbonated beverages are obvious bad-for-reflux drinks. Carbonated beverages are commercially acidified, hovering at a pH between 2 and 3. They will trigger irritation, burning, and LPR symptoms. Carbonation increases gases in the stomach, which leads to increased IAP, weakened LES muscles, and a splash of stomach content into the esophagus. Sugary drinks and juices are the perfect foods for gut bacteria to ferment.

Water is going to be your beverage of choice. If you're looking for something to flavor your water, add a few cucumber or melon slices. If you want a warm drink, add 1 teaspoon of grated fresh ginger to 1 cup of hot water, and sweeten with ½ teaspoon of pure maple syrup. Make an anti-inflammatory drink by warming lactose-free milk and mixing in 1 teaspoon of ground turmeric and 1 teaspoon of pure maple syrup. Even better, replace coffee and tea with a bowl of homemade bone broth that will soothe irritation in your throat and heal your gut.

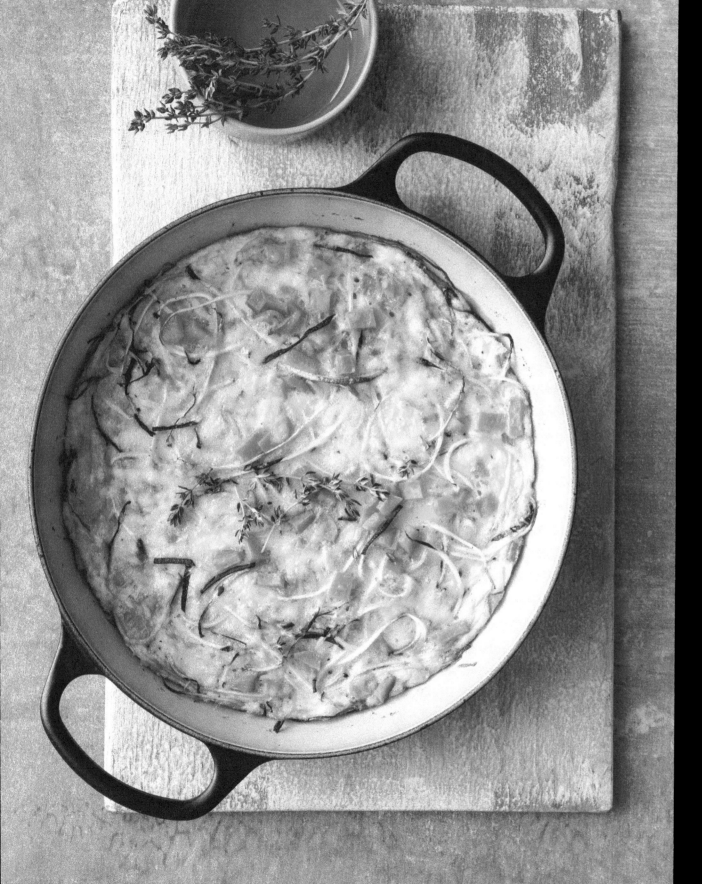

3

Different Meal Plans for Different Needs

Now that you know the big picture and your overall goals from the three different plans, it's time to dig deeper into the specific food lists.

Sorry, but this is not a magic-pill plan. For a time, you'll be eating in a different way than you're used to. But don't focus on what you lose; instead, focus on what you're gaining. Compared to how long you've been dealing with GERD or LPR and how severe your symptoms are, it's only a temporary sacrifice. Following the recipes in part 2 is much easier than trying to put together a plan on your own!

How to Make a Meal Plan Work for You

In the first two plans, you will remove foods that trigger and worsen acid reflux. In the third plan, you will methodically reintroduce some of the foods you eliminated to see if you're able to eat them again without triggering acid reflux symptoms. That will be your sign that healing has been accomplished.

Elimination plans can be challenging, so here are some tips to have healthy, healing meals ready at all times:

Plan ahead. Read the meal plan and recipes before going grocery shopping so you don't forget an ingredient. Organize your shopping list based on where the items are in the store. Don't forget breakfast and snacks.

Choose appealing recipes. If a meal does not sound appealing, skip it, and double up on other recipes that interest you more. You can swap one protein or vegetable for another so long as they are both in the "Enjoy" lists. In the recipes, I also give some suggestions for making substitutions.

Freeze extras. Buy freezer-safe glass containers to make your own microwavable meals. Stews, soups, meatballs, turkey burgers, baked chicken, and lamb kebabs freeze well. Freeze individual portions of cooked proteins in freezer-safe bags to quickly add to salads or have as a snack.

Take advantage of frozen produce. Frozen vegetables are okay! Grab a bag of frozen chopped spinach or trimmed green beans to steam or sauté when you are in a pinch for time.

Bulk cook. Cook enough for at least two meals. Cooking daily or multiple times a day is overwhelming, and you can't count on restaurant meals or takeouts during these plans. Double the recipes if other family members will be sharing your meals.

Cook two meals at once. Don't panic if no one in your household wants to eat like you do! There's no need to cook two different menus. Make the Halibut and Veggie Packets (page 136), and each person can add their own choice of vegetables and seasonings. Bake two trays of the Baked Chicken Tenders (page 144) side by side—one for you and another for everyone else with less restricted seasonings and spices. Roast your vegetables separately from the vegetables everyone else is eating.

THE THREE-DAY **STOP** PLAN

Here we go! The Three-Day STOP Plan is your jump start, with the goal of getting immediate relief in the fastest way possible. You won't eliminate as many foods as in the HEAL plan, so it's easier to follow. If you usually experience frequent and painful heartburn, you will notice a big difference in these three days. Just keep in mind that this plan doesn't dive into the underlying causes of heartburn, so you don't want your healing journey to end here.

In this plan, you will be removing extremely acidic foods and others known to be GERD and LPR irritants. This step is just a Band-Aid solution. While this seems to be against the long-term results you are trying to achieve, right now the cells that line the throat and esophagus need a break from acid so they can regenerate and heal. You don't want those lobster claws eating up your esophagus, and you certainly don't want to be in pain while you're discovering and solving the root of the problem.

Use the following food tables to navigate the Three-day STOP plan. Some of these foods will be taken out during the HEAL plan because they are high in FODMAPs. Make sure you check this table against the one in the HEAL plan so you don't buy too many vegetables or fruits that you won't be able to use after the three days are over.

For the fastest possible relief from your painful symptoms, eliminate these foods in the STOP plan:

ELIMINATE

FOOD OR FOOD GROUP	NOTEWORTHY INFORMATION
Alcoholic beverages	Relaxes LES, inflammatory
Caffeine	Relaxes LES
Carbonated beverages	Acidic, increases IAP, inflammatory

continued ▶

ELIMINATE (continued)

FOOD OR FOOD GROUP	NOTEWORTHY INFORMATION
Black and cayenne pepper, jalapeños, chiles, sriracha, hot sauce, spicy foods	Reflux trigger, irritant
Chocolate	Relaxes LES
Citrus fruits (clementine, grapefruit, lemon, lime, orange), berries, pineapples, grapes, peaches, nectarine, Granny Smith apples, cherries, kiwis	Acidic You may use a small squeeze of citrus juice or the grated zest on raw animal protein as a marinade, but avoid eating the fruit on its own.
Full-fat dairy, cream sauces, cheese sauces	Concentrated fat, keep food longer in the stomach, inflammatory
Fried foods	Reflux trigger, concentrated fat, keep food longer in the stomach, inflammatory
Processed and high-fat meats (bacon, high-fat burgers, high-fat red meat cuts, pepperoni, sausage)	Reflux trigger, concentrated fat, keep food longer in the stomach, inflammatory
Coffee, tea (black or green)	Reflux trigger You may be able to tolerate 1 cup decaffeinated.
Margarine, shortening	High in processed fat, acidic, inflammatory
Mint, peppermint	Reflux trigger
Green bell peppers	Reflux trigger

continued ▶

ELIMINATE (continued)

FOOD OR FOOD GROUP	NOTEWORTHY INFORMATION
Onions, garlic	Reflux trigger
Tomatoes, tomato sauce, tomato paste	Acidic, reflux trigger You may be able to tolerate 2 tablespoons of fresh tomato with starchy or protein-rich foods.
Vinegar	Acidic, irritant You may be able to tolerate a small amount on raw meats as a tenderizer.
Sugar	Inflammatory
Artificial sweeteners	Inflammatory, can disrupt natural gut pH

Now the good news! There are plenty of delicious foods that you can consume freely, without fear of your reflux symptoms coming back.

ENJOY

FOOD OR FOOD GROUP	EXAMPLES AND NOTEWORTHY INFORMATION
Non starchy vegetables	Artichokes (fresh or frozen, not canned), arugula, asparagus, bean sprouts, bok choy, broccoli, cabbage, cauliflower, celery, collard greens, cucumbers, eggplant, endive, escarole, fennel, ginger, kale, kelp (as a seasoning), leeks, lettuce, mushrooms, okra, spinach, string/green beans, thyme, yellow squash, zucchini

continued ▶

ENJOY (continued)

FOOD OR FOOD GROUP	EXAMPLES AND NOTEWORTHY INFORMATION
Root vegetables	Beets, butternut squash, carrots, parsnips, pumpkin, rutabagas, spaghetti squash, sweet potatoes, turnips, white potatoes
Fruit	Avocados (limit to ½ at a time due to fat content), bananas, cantaloupe, coconut (limit to ½ cup flesh or flakes due to fat content), dates, guava, honeydew, papaya, pears, red apples, watermelon
Protein	Chicken, eggs, fish, shellfish, turkey, lean beef, lean lamb, lean pork, tofu Choose ground beef that is at least 90 percent lean. Grill, steam, roast, bake, or sauté. Avoid frying.
Dairy or nondairy alternatives	Limit to 2 servings per day. A serving is 1 ounce hard cheese as a snack or garnish; or 1 cup yogurt, cottage cheese, or 2 percent milk; or 1 tablespoon half-and-half or sour cream. Nondairy alternatives such as coconut or almond milk
Nuts and seeds	Limit to 2 to 4 tablespoons per day of almonds, cashews, peanuts, pecans, pistachios, walnuts, chia seeds, flaxseed, hemp seeds, pumpkin seeds, or sunflower seeds. Limit to 2 tablespoons per day of peanut or almond butter; choose products without added oils, sugars, or salt.
Legumes	Beans, chickpeas, lentils, peas
Whole grains	Amaranth, barley, buckwheat, corn, millet, oats, quinoa, rice, rye, and whole wheat (bulgur, couscous, orzo, semolina, wheat-based pasta)

continued ▶

ENJOY (continued)

FOOD OR FOOD GROUP	EXAMPLES AND NOTEWORTHY INFORMATION
Oils	1 to 2 tablespoons per day of avocado oil, coconut oil, olive oil, grass-fed butter
Herbs and spices	Basil, cilantro, cinnamon, cumin, oregano, parsley, rosemary, thyme, turmeric, etc. Avoid hot spices, mint, and pepper.
Natural sweeteners	Limit to 1 to 3 teaspoons per day of agave nectar, honey, or pure maple syrup.
Other	Homemade bone broth without garlic or onion, black olives, coconut aminos (great soy-free replacement for soy sauce), miso, soy sauce, vanilla extract

You can stay on this plan longer if you need more time to adjust. But I do want you to get to the underlying causes as soon as possible, so don't stretch this phase for too long. Strive to start the HEAL plan within a week.

You do not need to eat a very low-fat diet on this plan. Do avoid greasy and fried foods, especially those breaded with flour, as flour can be a problem on its own. However, don't stress about using healthy oils or fats such as cold-pressed olive oil, coconut oil, nuts, and seeds. A small amount—say, a tablespoon of oil or an ounce of nuts—will add flavor and help you stay full.

You may be wondering about lemon juice and raw apple cider. These natural foods can stimulate digestion, which will ultimately help reduce acid reflux, but timing is key. The acid in lemon juice and vinegar can cause more damage as it travels down to the stomach. That's because pepsin, the protein-digesting enzyme produced by your stomach cells, is hanging out in your esophageal cells. It's going to get activated when acid is present and will irritate the esophagus lining. Remember that the stomach is coated by a mucous layer that protects it from acid and enzymes, while your esophagus is not.

The cells that line your digestive system typically regenerate every two to six days. When you stop stomach content from refluxing into the esophagus, which is the goal of the HEAL plan, your body will make healthy esophageal cells that don't have pepsin in them. You can expect to reset your esophagus and throat cells in just one week! After that point, your body will be more likely to tolerate lemon juice and raw apple cider vinegar. I include information on how to try them in the REINTRODUCE Plan. For now, though, avoiding them will improve your chances of success.

DAY 1

Breakfast: Banana-Flax Smoothie (page 70)

Morning Snack: 1 hard-boiled egg, 4 whole-grain crackers

Lunch: Pesto Grilled Cheese (page 128), ½ banana

Afternoon Snack: 1 celery stalk with 1 tablespoon peanut butter

Dinner: Ground Lamb and Lentil Chili (page 165)

DAY 2

Breakfast: Chia Breakfast Pudding with Cantaloupe (page 73)

Morning Snack: avocado toast (1 slice of whole-grain toast spread with ¼ avocado)

Lunch: Sirloin Steak Salad with Papaya Vinaigrette (page 157)

Afternoon Snack: 1 ounce almonds

Dinner: Maple-Glazed Salmon (page 139), Artichoke Purée (page 97)

DAY 3

Breakfast: Baked Avocado and Egg (page 85)

Morning snack: Turkey-Wrapped Melon (page 178)

Lunch: Italian Vegetable Soup (page 111)

Afternoon Snack: 1 cup cantaloupe balls

Dinner: Baked Chicken Tenders (page 144), ¼ cup steamed broccoli, Sweet Potato French Fries (page 96)

SNACK IDEAS

- 1 hard-boiled egg
- 1 celery stalk with 2 tablespoons peanut butter
- 1 cup cantaloupe balls
- avocado toast: 1 piece of whole-grain toast spread with ¼ avocado
- 3 cups air-popped popcorn

THE FOUR-WEEK **HEAL** PLAN

By now you should be feeling relief from your symptoms, which is great, but you're not quite there yet. This plan is the most important plan in the book, because if you don't solve the root of the problem, you will always battle acid reflux by eliminating acidic foods or depending on acid-blocking medication—or else suffer from painful and serious consequences.

As we discussed earlier, the root cause of acid reflux is *not* excess acid. Fermentation of poorly digested carbohydrates in the stomach and small intestine yields a large volume of gases. These gases push open the LES muscles that separate the stomach from the esophagus, causing the stomach content, including HCl and pepsin, to reflux upward. Hydrochloric acid and pepsin are not bad for you, except when they're in the wrong place!

The goal of the four-week HEAL plan is to eliminate the foods that contribute to fermentation while still avoiding acidic foods. The plan combines the three-day low-acid STOP plan with a low-FODMAP diet. While this is more challenging, I find that the combination helps my patients get the best results. And that's what I want for you, too.

You're going to continue to eliminate the same foods you did in the STOP plan. You'll find the list on page 38. The new piece is eliminating foods that are high in FODMAPs. They are not acidic, and many of them are healthy, anti-inflammatory foods, but since they have the fibers that tend to make delicious food for gut bacteria, resulting in too much gas and IAP, you're going to remove them for the next four weeks.

You can expect to notice improvement in just two weeks on the plan. But don't rush into reintroductions just yet. Most people need the full four weeks for the results to settle in. You may better tolerate acidic foods, such as pineapple and berries, toward the end of the plan as the lining of your esophagus heals. Dietary acid will no longer bother you because pepsin has not damaged the new cells. For this reason, you might be tempted to loosen up the diet, but do your absolute best to stick to it. Four weeks may seem like a really long time, but compared to how long you've been dealing with your symptoms, it's a short time and absolutely worth the effort.

The following tables are similar to the one for the STOP plan, with one exception. **Note that in the second table, which lists foods that can be enjoyed on the HEAL plan, certain foods are listed in boldface. These foods contain moderate amounts of FODMAPs, and as such, they should be eaten in limited amounts when applicable.** The suggested serving sizes are provided.

ELIMINATE

FOOD GROUP	FOODS	NOTEWORTHY INFORMATION
Foods that relax the LES	Alcoholic beverages	Alcoholic beverages are also inflammatory.
	Caffeine	
	Chocolate	
Acidic foods	Carbonated beverages	Carbonated beverages also increase IAP and inflammation.
	Citrus fruits (clementine, grapefruit, lemon, lime, orange), berries, pineapples, grapes, peaches, nectarine, Granny Smith apples, cherries, kiwis	You may use a small squeeze of citrus juice or the grated zest on raw animal protein as a marinade, but avoid eating the fruit on its own.
	Vinegar	You may be able to tolerate a small amount of vinegar on raw meats as a tenderizer.
	Tomatoes, tomato sauce, tomato paste	You may be able to tolerate 2 tablespoons of fresh tomato with starchy or protein-rich foods.

continued ▶

ELIMINATE (continued)

FOOD GROUP	FOODS	NOTEWORTHY INFORMATION
Fatty foods	Full-fat dairy, cream sauces, cheese sauces	Concentrated fats keep food longer in the stomach and are also inflammatory.
	Fried foods	
	Processed and high-fat meats (bacon, high-fat burgers, high-fat red meat cuts, pepperoni, sausage)	
	Margarine, shortening	Margarine and shortening are high in processed fats, acidic, and inflammatory.
Common reflux triggers	Coffee, tea (black or green)	You may be able to tolerate 1 cup decaffeinated.
	Mint, peppermint	
	Green bell peppers	
	Onions, garlic	

continued ▶

ELIMINATE (continued)

FOOD GROUP	FOODS	NOTEWORTHY INFORMATION
Inflammatory foods	Artificial sweeteners	Artificial sweeteners can also disrupt natural gut pH.
	Sugar	
Non starchy vegetables	Asparagus, cabbage, cauliflower, leeks, mushrooms	High in FODMAPs
Root vegetables	Beets	High in FODMAPs
Fruit	Dates, guava, papaya, pears, red apples, watermelon	High in FODMAPs
Protein	Soft or silken tofu	High in FODMAPs
Dairy	Cottage cheese, cream cheese, feta cheese, goat cheese, sour cream	High in FODMAPs
Nuts	Cashews, pistachios	High in FODMAPs
Legumes	Avoid all beans, chickpeas, lentils, peas	High in FODMAPs Exception: Canned chickpeas and lentils may be okay in small amounts (see next table)

continued ▶

ELIMINATE (continued)

FOOD GROUP	FOODS	NOTEWORTHY INFORMATION
Whole grains	Barley, rye, whole wheat (bulgur, couscous, orzo, semolina, wheat-based pasta)	High in FODMAPs
Other	Soy sauce	May contain FODMAPs such as onion, garlic, and wheat

ENJOY

FOOD OR FOOD GROUP	EXAMPLES AND NOTEWORTHY INFORMATION
Non starchy vegetables	Arugula, bean sprouts, bok choy, **broccoli (limit to ½ cup), celery (limit to 1 stalk),** collard greens, cucumbers, eggplant, endive, escarole, fennel, ginger, kale, kelp (as a seasoning), lettuce, okra, spinach, string/green beans, thyme, yellow squash, zucchini
Root vegetables	**Butternut squash (limit to ½ cup),** carrots, parsnip, **pumpkin (limit to 1 cup),** rutabagas, spaghetti squash, sweet potato (limit to ½ cup) turnips, white potatoes
Fruit	**Avocados (limit to ⅛),** bananas, cantaloupe, **coconut (limit to ½ cup fresh or flakes),** honeydew
Protein	Chicken, eggs, fish, shellfish, turkey, lean beef, lean lamb, lean pork, firm, drained tofu Choose ground beef that is at least 90 percent lean. Grill, steam, roast, bake, or sauté. Avoid frying.

continued ▶

ENJOY (continued)

FOOD OR FOOD GROUP	EXAMPLES AND NOTEWORTHY INFORMATION
Dairy or nondairy alternatives	Limit to 2 servings per day. A serving is **1 ounce hard cheese** as a snack or garnish, **1 tablespoon half-and-half, or 1 cup lactose-free dairy including yogurt, cottage cheese, or 2 percent milk.** Nondairy alternatives such as **almond milk (limit to 1 cup) or coconut milk (limit to ½ cup)**
Nuts and seeds	Limit to **2 tablespoons per day of almonds (10 pieces),** peanuts, pecans, walnuts, chia seeds, flaxseed, hemp seeds, pumpkin seeds, sunflower seeds. Limit to **1 tablespoon almond butter** or 2 tablespoons peanut butter per day; choose products without added oils, sugars, or salt.
Legumes	**You may be able to tolerate ¼ cup canned chickpeas or ½ cup canned lentils.**
Whole grains	Amaranth, buckwheat, millet, oats, quinoa, rice **You may have corn flour or corn tortilla. Limit corn kernels to ½ cup per day.**
Oils	1 to 2 tablespoons per day of avocado oil, coconut oil, olive oil, grass-fed butter
Herbs and spices	Basil, cilantro, cinnamon, cumin, oregano, parsley, rosemary, thyme, turmeric, etc. Avoid hot spices, mint, and pepper.
Natural sweeteners	You may have 1 to 3 teaspoons per day of pure maple syrup.

continued ▶

ENJOY (continued)

FOOD OR FOOD GROUP	EXAMPLES AND NOTEWORTHY INFORMATION
Other	Homemade bone broth without garlic or onion, black olives, coconut aminos (great soy-free replacement for soy sauce), miso, vanilla extract

SPECIAL HEALING FOODS

Certain foods help the lining of your digestive tract heal. Many of them come in a concentrated dose as dietary supplements. However, in this book we focus on food, as it is better to consult with your health care provider when it comes to supplements.

Ginger. My favorite gut-healing food is ginger. It improves gastric emptying, which is how fast your stomach empties its content to the small intestine. As acid, pepsin, and bile move farther away from the esophagus, reflux is less likely to happen.

Bone broth. Bone broth contains collagen, a protein found in the connective tissue of animals and the most abundant protein in the human body. It is rich in the amino acid glutamine, which helps protect, nourish, and repair the cells of the digestive tract. Drink a cup of Poultry Broth (page 195) each day as a warm soothing beverage in place of coffee. Use the broth in soups and stews. Replace some of the oils in your old recipes with a few tablespoons of broth.

Probiotic foods. Probiotic foods help restore your gut flora balance. This is important because problems with digestion and bacterial overgrowth deep in the gut can trigger GERD and acid reflux. Yogurt contains *Lactobacillus* species, the predominant type of bacteria in the small intestine. This species also helps break down undigested carbohydrates without producing a lot of gas.

Lactose-free yogurt. As lactose is easily fermentable and digestive pains in some people, it's best to eat lactose-free yogurt. Make sure the label states that it contains "active" cultures, and choose plain varieties without added sugars or preservatives. If you want your yogurt to be sweet, add a teaspoon of pure maple syrup or mix in some chopped cantaloupe or banana. If lactose-free yogurt is not available where you shop, stick to a small amount of Greek yogurt or kefir yogurt, if you can tolerate them. If you have IBS or other advanced digestive conditions, you will probably need a therapeutic dose of probiotic supplements. Your health care provider can direct you to the best types and concentrations for your specific health need.

Fermented foods. You may be wondering about fermented foods such as sauerkraut, kimchi, and kombucha. They are excellent sources of healthy bacteria, but their high acidity can trigger heartburn symptoms if you eat them early on in the plan. Wait until you complete the HEAL plan and then experiment with introducing them.

Omega-3 fatty acids. Foods high in omega-3 fatty acids are anti-inflammatory. While some omega-3 fatty acids are found in plants such as walnuts and flaxseeds, marine-based omega-3s are needed for reducing inflammation. That's because your body may not be able to convert the plant-based omega-3s to the potent anti-inflammatory omega-3s that only come from marine sources. I include several fish recipes to help you get omega-3s naturally from foods such as salmon and tuna. Fish oil supplements are readily available in many retail stores, and you can find algae-based omega-3s if you want a vegetarian option. Except for people on blood thinners or those at risk of prostate cancer, fish oil supplements are generally considered safe. Look for high-quality products and consult with your health care provider.

Aloe vera. Aloe vera is another excellent healing food. You may have seen aloe drinks, but they typically contain too much sugar and preservatives. Use it naturally by adding aloe gel to smoothies. Cut a 2-inch piece of aloe stem, remove the hard green part, and add the clear gooey material to your smoothie.

Pineapple and papaya. These fruits contain natural enzymes that help improve digestion and reduce fermentation of carbohydrates. Bromelain enzyme is found in the flesh but is concentrated in the stem and core of pineapples. Papain enzyme comes from papaya. Pineapples are too acidic and papayas contain fructose, so both are off limits in the HEAL plan. However, when your acid symptoms improve and you move to the REINTRODUCE plan, these should be among the first foods to try. Start with a small amount, about ¼ cup. Digestive enzymes also come in supplement form, but the quality and potency is different from one product to another. A dietitian can help you determine if you need one and recommend the best type for your symptoms.

WEEK 1

Monday
Breakfast: Sweet Melon Smoothie (page 71)
Morning Snack: Deviled Egg (page 172)
Lunch: Fried Egg Sandwich (page 129)
Afternoon Snack: ¾ cup lactose-free plain nonfat yogurt, ½ banana
Dinner: Turkey Meatloaf Muffin (page 150), Mashed Potatoes (page 101), 1 cup steamed broccoli

Tuesday
Breakfast: Fruit and Yogurt Parfait (page 74)
Morning Snack: Baked Potato Chips (page 176)
Lunch: Chicken Noodle Soup (page 143)
Afternoon Snack: Cucumber Rounds with Shrimp Salad (page 175)
Dinner: Beef Tacos (page 161)

Wednesday
Breakfast: Sweet Melon Smoothie (page 71)
Morning Snack: 1 slice gluten-free toast with 1 teaspoon peanut butter
Lunch: Soba Noodles with Peanut Butter Sauce (page 121)
Afternoon Snack: Cinnamon-Sugar Popcorn (page 174)

Dinner: Baked Chicken Tenders (page 144), Green Beans Amandine (page 98)

Thursday
Breakfast: Toads in a Hole (page 82)
Morning Snack: Carrots with Herbed Yogurt Dip (page 177)
Lunch: Creamy Pumpkin Soup (page 112)
Afternoon Snack: Grated Carrot and Raisin Salad (page 179)
Dinner: Steamer Clams with Fennel (page 135), 1 slice gluten-free whole-grain toast

Friday
Breakfast: Corn Porridge with Maple and Raisins (page 77)
Morning Snack: 1 ounce pepitas (hulled pumpkin seeds)
Lunch: Pesto Grilled Cheese (page 128)
Afternoon Snack: 2 slices deli turkey and carrot sticks
Dinner: Maple-Glazed Salmon (page 139), steamed carrots

Saturday
Breakfast: Salmon and Egg Scramble (page 87)
Morning Snack: Banana and Melon Salad (page 188)
Lunch: Fisherman's Stew (page 142)
Afternoon Snack: Spiced Walnuts (page 173)
Dinner: Pho with Beef and Zucchini Noodles (page 155)

continued ▶

Sunday

Breakfast: Banana Pancakes
(page 80)

Morning Snack: Zucchini Hummus
(page 93)

Lunch: Easy Turkey Burgers
(page 148), carrot sticks

Afternoon Snack: ¼ cup lactose-free
plain nonfat yogurt, ½ banana

Dinner: Inside-Out Cabbage
Rolls (page 158), ½ cup
steamed spinach

WEEK 2

Monday

Breakfast: Raisin Cornmeal
Pancakes (page 78)

Morning Snack: Turkey-Wrapped
Melon (page 178)

Lunch: One-Pot Chicken Stew
(page 147)

Afternoon Snack: Baked Potato
Chips (page 176)

Dinner: Turkey and Spinach Rollatini
(page 151), ½ baked potato with
1 tablespoon grass-fed butter

Tuesday

Breakfast: Banana-Flax Smoothie
(page 70)

Morning Snack: carrot sticks with
Zucchini Hummus (page 93)

Lunch: Easy Tuna Melt (page 138)

Afternoon Snack: Peanut Butter
and Carob Balls (page 180)

Dinner: Shepherd's Pie Muffins
(page 163)

Wednesday

Breakfast: Fruit and Yogurt Parfait
(page 74)

Morning Snack: 1 banana

Lunch: Hamburger Stew (page 160)

Afternoon Snack: Deviled Egg
(page 172)

Dinner: Crab Cakes with Tartar
Sauce (page 132), 1 cup steamed
broccoli

Thursday

Breakfast: Turkey and Egg Breakfast
Sandwich (page 83)

Morning Snack: Spiced Walnuts
(page 173)

Lunch: Vegetable and Tofu Fried
Rice (page 123)

Afternoon Snack: Melon with Ginger
Dipping Sauce (page 182)

Dinner: Herb-Crusted Lamb Chops
(page 166), Green Beans Amandine (page 98)

Friday

Breakfast: Sweet Melon Smoothie
(page 71)

Morning Snack: 1 cup honeydew
melon balls

Lunch: Patty Melt Soup (page 156)

Afternoon Snack: Spinach and Dill
Dip (page 92)

Dinner: Asian Veggie and Tofu
Stir-Fry (page 120)

continued ▶

Saturday

Breakfast: Puffy Omelet (page 89)

Morning Snack: Olive Tapenade (page 95), 4 gluten-free crackers

Lunch: Zucchini Ribbons with Parmesan Cream Sauce (page 119)

Afternoon Snack: Cinnamon-Sugar Popcorn (page 174)

Dinner: Tilapia with Cantaloupe Salsa (page 137), ¼ cup steamed brown rice

Sunday

Breakfast: French Toast (page 79)

Morning Snack: ¼ cup lactose-free plain nonfat yogurt, ½ banana

Lunch: Fish Tacos with Guacamole (page 141)

Afternoon Snack: Turkey-Wrapped Melon (page 178)

Dinner: Oven-Fried Chicken (page 145), steamed carrots, Baked Potato Chips (page 176)

WEEK 3

Monday

Breakfast: Corn Porridge with Maple and Raisins (page 77)

Morning Snack: Peanut Butter and Banana Spread with Ginger (page 181) with carrot sticks

Lunch: Cream of Broccoli Soup (page 113)

Afternoon Snack: Peanut Butter and Carob Balls (page 180)

Dinner: Lamb Meatballs with Lemon Yogurt Sauce (page 164), 1 cup salad greens with Creamy Herbed Dressing (page 200)

Tuesday

Breakfast: Banana Pancakes (page 80)

Morning Snack: 1 slice gluten-free whole-grain toast or 4 gluten-free whole-grain crackers, spread with ⅛ avocado

Lunch: Brown Rice and Peanut Lettuce Wraps (page 122)

Afternoon Snack: 1 ounce sunflower seeds or pepitas (hulled pumpkin seeds)

Dinner: Roasted Lamb Chops with Chimichurri (page 167), Mashed Potatoes (page 101), steamed carrots

Wednesday

Breakfast: Toads in a Hole (page 82)

Morning Snack: Yogurt and Melon Ice Pops (page 185)

Lunch: Fisherman's Stew (page 142)

Afternoon Snack: Baked Potato Chips (page 176)

Dinner: Grilled Eggplant Burgers (page 127) with Lemon Yogurt Sauce (page 199), carrot sticks

continued ▶

Thursday

Breakfast: Sweet Melon Smoothie (page 71)

Morning Snack: hard-boiled egg, 2 tablespoons raisins

Lunch: Broccoli and Cheese Baked Potato (page 115)

Afternoon Snack: ½ banana, 1 ounce pepitas (hulled pumpkin seeds)

Dinner: Halibut and Veggie Packets (page 136)

Friday

Breakfast: Spinach Frittata (page 86)

Morning Snack: Turkey-Wrapped Melon (page 178)

Lunch: Brown Rice and Tofu with Kale (page 125)

Afternoon Snack: Zucchini Hummus (page 93) with carrot sticks

Dinner: Miso-Glazed Scallops (page 133), steamed spinach

Saturday

Breakfast: 1 egg your way, Sweet Potato Hash (page 81)

Morning Snack: Spiced Walnuts (page 173)

Lunch: Fried Egg Sandwich (page 129)

Afternoon Snack: 1 banana

Dinner: Maple-Glazed Salmon (page 139), Sweet Potato French Fries (page 96), Green Beans Amandine (page 98)

Sunday

Breakfast: Salmon and Egg Scramble (page 87)

Morning Snack: Melon with Ginger Dipping Sauce (page 182)

Lunch: Easy Tuna Melt (page 138)

Afternoon Snack: 1 banana

Dinner: Breaded Crispy Shrimp (page 134), carrot sticks

WEEK 4

Monday

Breakfast: French Toast (page 79)

Morning Snack: Deviled Egg (page 172)

Lunch: Pasta with Walnut Pesto (page 117)

Afternoon Snack: ¼ cup lactose-free plain nonfat yogurt, 1 cup melon balls

Dinner: Quick Chicken and Veggie Stir-Fry (page 146), ¼ cup steamed brown rice

Tuesday

Breakfast: Banana-Flax Smoothie (page 70)

Morning Snack: Cinnamon-Sugar Popcorn (page 174)

Lunch: Turkey Meatballs (page 149), ¼ cup steamed brown rice

Afternoon Snack: Yogurt and Melon Ice Pops (page 185)

Dinner: Seasoned Tofu with Chimichurri (page 126), steamed zucchini

continued ▶

Wednesday

Breakfast: Raisin Cornmeal Pancakes (page 78)

Morning Snack: Peanut Butter and Carob Balls (page 180)

Lunch: Vegetable Beef Soup (page 154)

Afternoon Snack: 1 slice gluten-free whole-grain toast spread with ⅛ avocado

Dinner: Sweet Potato and Corn Stew (page 114)

Thursday

Breakfast: Toads in a Hole (page 82)

Morning Snack: 1 cup melon balls

Lunch: Chicken Noodle Soup (page 143)

Afternoon Snack: Peanut Butter and Banana Spread with Ginger (page 181) on 6 gluten-free whole-grain crackers

Dinner: Grilled Eggplant Burgers (page 127) with Lemon Yogurt Sauce (page 199), carrot sticks

Friday

Breakfast: Fruit and Yogurt Parfait (page 74)

Morning Snack: Deviled Eggs (page 172)

Lunch: Quick Chicken and Veggie Stir-Fry (page 146)

Afternoon Snack: Spiced Walnuts (page 173)

Dinner: Fish Tacos with Guacamole (page 141)

Saturday

Breakfast: 1 egg your way, Turkey Breakfast Sausage (page 84)

Morning Snack: 1 slice gluten-free whole-grain toast topped with ½ banana

Lunch: Easy Tuna Melt (page 138)

Afternoon Snack: Yogurt and Melon Ice Pops (page 185)

Dinner: Cream of Broccoli Soup (page 113)

Sunday

Breakfast: Puffy Omelet (page 89)

Morning Snack: Banana and Melon Salad (page 188)

Lunch: Pho with Beef and Zucchini Noodles (page 155)

Afternoon Snack: Peanut Butter Cookies (page 190)

Dinner: Cod with Cantaloupe Salsa (page 206), Quinoa Pilaf (page 102)

THE FOUR-WEEK
REINTRODUCE PLAN

In this plan, we are going to slowly introduce foods that are high in FODMAPs and foods that are acidic. By now, you should be feeling great. No more heartburn or acid reflux, no more coughing or lump sensation, and if you had bloating or stomach pain, it should be gone as well.

Some of my patients who feel amazing after the HEAL plan do not want to reintroduce the foods they eliminated. While it might be tempting to stick with the diet because it makes you feel better, it is not a sustainable lifestyle. Several of the eliminated foods provide your body with healthy fiber, antioxidants, vitamins, and minerals, so we want to slowly bring them back. Your digestive system should be able to handle them well now.

To introduce a new food, follow this sequence:

- On day 1, eat a small portion of the food. The amount for each food is specified in the following tables.
- On day 2, eat a larger portion of the food.
- On days 3 to 5, reset by going back to the HEAL plan.
- On day 6, introduce a small portion of another food.
- Repeat.

It may take more than four weeks to go through all the foods suggested for introduction. That's okay. Choose what you miss the most first—but not processed foods or soda! While you may expect foods from the same group to cause the same reaction, I've found that not to be the case with my patients. For example, you may be able to tolerate garlic, but not onion or celery, even though they are all in the fructan group. (Refer the table on page 23 for the different FODMAP groups.) That's why I encourage you to try foods individually and not make a generalization. However, if a particular food caused a severe acid reflux reaction, don't rush into introducing others in the same group just yet.

Add foods slowly to avoid overwhelming your digestive system and ending up with sudden heartburn. If a small portion doesn't trigger any symptoms, you can move on with confidence to a larger portion. But if the small portion increased reflux or caused any other undesirable symptom, don't proceed to the large portion. Skip it and go straight into the reset days. The reset days will help you separate the effect of one food from another. To figure out which foods might be triggers, don't try a new food until you are completely free of heartburn or other symptoms.

The number of days needed to reset will vary from one person to another. The idea is to wait until one food is completely out of your system before adding another. This will depend on your own transit time, the time it takes food to pass through your entire digestive tract. On average, it takes 33 to 47 hours for a food to be excreted. Men have a faster transit time than women. Certain conditions such as gastroparesis, hypothyroidism, and nerve damage slow down digestion. You may need a longer time to process food if you have one of those conditions.

Pick a food from the tables and stick to the given amount. Note any heartburn, acid reflux, or other symptoms, if any, in the space provided in the table. If an acidic food such as tomato triggers heartburn, don't add another acidic food, such as an orange—you may not be ready for them yet. In the next section, I will talk about what to do if you continue to experience acid reflux despite following the plan.

When you introduce a new food, have it as a snack or add it to an individual portion of a recipe rather than incorporating it into a big batch. You don't want to waste time and ingredients if it turns out you can't eat it again.

If you experience acid reflux when reintroducing a food, you can occasionally use baking soda to get immediate relief. Baking soda contains sodium bicarbonate, which is a base that neutralizes acid. In fact, the pancreas produces sodium bicarbonate regularly to neutralize the acidic stomach content when it arrives at the intestine. Mix ¼ teaspoon baking soda with ½ cup water and drink it when you experience heartburn. This should only be a temporary fix! Don't take more than 1½ teaspoons of baking soda a day, and don't use baking soda for more than two weeks, because too much baking soda can lead to acid rebound, which means your stomach overproduces acid as a response. Also, be aware that baking soda is concentrated in sodium and therefore not a good option if you're on a sodium-restricted diet. You can try a commercial product such as Tums or Alka-Seltzer to get through a flare-up. Hopefully, with this plan, you will not need to use any of them.

Here are some suggestions for types and amounts of foods to try for the small and large reintroduction challenges. You can try eating the test food alone, or incorporate it into one of the suggested recipes. (Of course, there are many other recipes you can use as well; check the recipe's REINTRODUCE tip to make sure it is suitable.)

FOOD, FODMAP CATEGORY (PORTION)		
SUGGESTED RECIPES	**PHYSICAL REACTIONS**	**SAFE FOOD?**
Garlic, fructan (Small amount: 1 clove, Large amount: 3 cloves)		
See the REINTRODUCE tips for these recipes: Zucchini Hummus (page 93) Soba Noodles with Peanut Butter Sauce (page 121) Oven-Fried Chicken (page 145)		Y / N
Onion, fructan (Small amount: 1 small onion, Large amount: 2 or 3 onions)		
See the REINTRODUCE tips for these recipes: Italian Vegetable Soup (page 111) Butternut Risotto (page 124) Crab Cakes with Tartar Sauce (page 132)		Y / N

continued ▶

FOOD, FODMAP CATEGORY (PORTION)		
SUGGESTED RECIPES	PHYSICAL REACTIONS	SAFE FOOD?
Avocado, polyol (Small amount: ½ avocado, Large amount: 1 avocado)		
Baked Avocado and Egg (page 85)	_____	
Fish Tacos with Guacamole (page 141): increase amount of guacamole	_____ _____ _____	Y / N
Mushroom, polyol (Small amount: ½ cup raw, Large amount: 1 cup raw)		
Hamburger Stroganoff with Zucchini Noodles (page 159)	_____ _____	
Quick Chicken and Veggie Stir-Fry (page 146): add 1 cup mushrooms	_____ _____ _____	Y / N
Celery, fructan (Small amount: 2 stalks, Large amount: 3 or more stalks)		
Chicken Noodle Soup (page 143): add 2 chopped celery stalks when cooking onions	_____ _____ _____ _____	Y / N
Honey, fructose (Small amount: 1 teaspoon, Large amount: 1 tablespoon)		
Turkey and Egg Breakfast Sandwich (page 83): see REINTRODUCE tip	_____ _____	
Roasted Honey-Ginger Carrots (page 103)	_____ _____	Y / N

REINTRODUCE

continued ▶

FOOD, FODMAP CATEGORY (PORTION)		
SUGGESTED RECIPES	**PHYSICAL REACTIONS**	**SAFE FOOD?**
Red apple or pear, fructose, fructan, and polyol (Small amount: ½ fruit, Large amount: 1 fruit)		
Fruit and Yogurt Parfait (page 74): see REINTRODUCE tip Apple Compote Smoothie (page 75)	_____ _____ _____ _____	Y / N
Milk or yogurt (regular, not lactose-free), lactose (Small amount: ½ cup, Large amount: 1 cup)		
Fruit and Yogurt Parfait (page 74) Mashed Potatoes (page 101): use regular milk	_____ _____ _____ _____	Y / N
Wheat-based pasta, fructan (Small amount: ½ cup, Large amount: 1 cup)		
Chicken Noodle Soup (page 143): use regular spaghetti Pho with Beef and Zucchini Noodles (page 155): use angel hair pasta instead of zucchini noodles	_____ _____ _____	Y / N

REINTRODUCING FOODS THAT ARE ACIDIC
OR TRADITIONALLY KNOWN AS REFLUX TRIGGERS

Here are some suggestions for types and amounts of foods to try for the small and large reintroduction challenges. You can try eating the test food alone, or incorporate it into one of the suggested recipes.

FOOD (PORTION)		
SUGGESTED RECIPES	**PHYSICAL REACTIONS**	**SAFE FOOD?**
Clementine (Small amount: 1 fruit, Large amount: 2 fruits)		
Banana and Melon Salad (page 188): add 2 clementines in sections	_____ _____ _____	Y / N
Orange (Small amount: ½ fruit, Large amount: 1 fruit)		
Banana and Melon Salad (page 188): add orange sections Chia Breakfast Pudding with Cantaloupe (page 73): replace cantaloupe with orange sections	_____ _____ _____	Y / N
Pineapple (Small amount: ½ cup, Large amount: 1 cup)		
Chia Breakfast Pudding with Cantaloupe (page 73): see REINTRODUCE tip	_____ _____ _____	Y / N

continued ▶

FOOD (PORTION)		
SUGGESTED RECIPES	**PHYSICAL REACTIONS**	**SAFE FOOD?**
Tomato (Small amount: ½ cup fresh, Large amount: ½ cup or more tomato sauce)		
Grilled Eggplant Burgers with Lemon Yogurt Sauce (pages 127 and 199): see REINTRODUCE tip	_____ _____	Y / N
Halibut and Veggie Packets (page 136): see REINTRODUCE tip	_____ _____	
Berries (Small amount: ½ cup, Large amount: 1 cup)		
Raisin Cornmeal Pancakes (page 78): see REINTRODUCE tip	_____ _____ _____	Y / N
Sauerkraut (Small amount: 1 tablespoon, Large amount: ¼ cup)		
N/A	_____ _____	Y / N
Raw apple cider vinegar (Small amount: 1 teaspoon mixed with ½ cup water, Large amount: 1 tablespoon mixed with ½ cup water)		
Creamy Herbed Dressing (page 200): whisk in 1 tablespoon apple cider vinegar	_____ _____ _____	Y / N

continued ▶

FOOD (PORTION)		
SUGGESTED RECIPES	**PHYSICAL REACTIONS**	**SAFE FOOD?**
Lemon juice (Small amount: 1 tablespoon freshly squeezed lemon juice with 1 cup water, Large amount: 2 tablespoons freshly squeezed lemon juice with 1 cup water)		
Walnut-Basil Pesto (page 201): add 2 tablespoons lemon juice		
Oregano and Parsley Chimichurri (page 205): add 2 tablespoons lemon juice	_____	Y / N
Bell pepper (Small amount: ½ pepper, Large amount: 1 pepper)		
Beef Tacos (page 161): see REINTRODUCE tip	_____	Y / N
Coffee, tea (caffeinated) (1 cup)		
N/A	_____	Y / N
Chocolate, dark (Small amount: 1 ounce, Large amount: 2 ounces)		
Peanut Butter Cookies (page 190): add 1 teaspoon dark chocolate chips to each cookie	_____	Y / N
Peppermint tea (Small amount: ½ cup, Large amount: 1 cup)		
N/A	_____	Y / N

Coping with Cravings and Dietary Changes

Diet changes are not easy. They push you out of your comfort zone, and you may be tempted to give in to cravings. Please don't. You are already well on your way to healing your acid reflux. Let's talk about coping with emotional and physical cravings.

Remember that this is a transitional phase, and you will not need to restrict your food forever. The damage may have been happening for years, so give your digestive lining a few weeks to heal and reset. Think positive. Focus on the results you want and the pain and discomfort you are freeing yourself from. Imagine the new healthy cells your body is producing as beautiful blossoming flowers, thanks to every healthy choice you make. Food is your medicine. Eat to live; don't live to eat.

Planning ahead will help prevent impulse food decisions that might interfere with your progress. Plan all your meals and snacks. Cook during the weekend. Grab a snack to take with you when you run errands. Pack enough food to take to work. Eat every four hours so you don't get too hungry. At meals, eat protein and a moderate amount of fat to stay feeling full longer.

Remember to be mindful when you eat. Being present in the moment and focusing on your food will help you feel more satisfied. It also helps you slow down and chew food thoroughly, which is necessary to prevent indigestion and reflux.

If you do have a craving, wait before you respond to it. Instead of immediately running to your refrigerator or pantry, first drink a cup of water. Then sit comfortably in a quiet place. Breathe deeply and slowly for five minutes. Distract yourself with calming and relaxing thoughts. You may realize that you're not hungry after all. Your craving may be emotional because you are procrastinating about a boring task that you need to complete, or you may be sleepy and just need a short nap!

If the craving persists, it may be true physical hunger. Review your food lists and pick something that will not throw you off track. Ideally, your kitchen is stocked with foods that are allowed on the plans. The more you practice slowing down and being mindful, the better you'll get at managing cravings.

Cooking Wisely to Prevent Acid Reflux

It can be tough to say good-bye to your favorite comfort foods. But with some creative cooking methods and the recipes in this book, it's still possible to enjoy your meals without suffering the consequences.

- Instead of frying, bake, grill, or roast your foods. For example, the Baked Chicken Tenders recipe (page 144) replaces fried chicken. You can make oven-baked potatoes instead of deep-frying them.
- Use flavorful extra-virgin olive oil, coconut oil, or even grass-fed butter to flavor your food. You don't need a lot of fat to enjoy your meals. Just a little adds flavor. Use just enough to prevent burning (lowering the heat also helps).
- When you make chicken or beef bone broth, cook a large batch and save the extra in the freezer in either 1-cup or 2-cup glass jars. When you want to use some, thawing it overnight in the refrigerator is best.
- If you have access to a microwave and a refrigerator or freezer at work, leave some of your food staples and supplies there.
- Store all the ingredients you can eat during the plan in a certain cabinet or container in your kitchen. Alternatively, move aside everything you can't eat, or give it to a friend.
- Ginger adds so much flavor to meals and comes in extra handy because you will not be using garlic or onion. You can also grate a ½-inch cube of peeled ginger and add it to warm water to drink in the morning or between meals.

Kitchen Equipment and Pantry List

The following equipment and pantry items play a key role in the recipes in this book. All are affordable and easy to find. If for some reason you are unable to find the items locally, most are available online.

ESSENTIAL EQUIPMENT

Pots and Pans

- 3 nonstick skillets (8-inch, 10-inch, and 12-inch)
- Large soup pot (7 to 9 quarts)
- 3 saucepans (3 to 6 quarts)
- Ovenproof skillet (12-inch)
- 2 rimmed 9-by-13-inch baking sheets
- Loaf pan
- 6-cup muffin tin
- Square baking pan

Mixing and Cutting

- Chef's knife
- Paring knife
- Wooden spoons
- Silicone scrapers
- Spatula
- Whisk
- Small, medium, and large mixing bowls

Measuring

- Full set of measuring cups
- Full set of measuring spoons
- 2-cup liquid measure

Miscellaneous equipment

- Rasp-style grater
- Box grater
- Colander
- Vegetable peeler
- Ladle
- Instant-read thermometer
- Silicone brush
- Meat mallet
- Melon baller
- Ice pop mold
- Eggbeater
- Parchment paper
- Aluminum foil
- Toothpicks

Other

- Blender or small food processor
- Indoor or outdoor grill or stove top grill pan

PANTRY STAPLES

Stocking your pantry will make it easier to prepare all the recipes in this cook-book, even when you're in a hurry. Keep the following staples on hand.

Herbs, Spices, and Flavorings

- Allspice, ground
- Cinnamon, ground
- Cloves, ground
- Coconut aminos
- Coriander, ground
- Cumin, ground
- Dill, dried
- Fish sauce
- Ginger, ground
- Miso
- Mustard, Dijon
- Mustard, ground
- Nutmeg, ground
- Oregano, dried
- Sea salt
- Soy sauce, gluten-free (tamari)
- Tarragon, dried
- Thyme, dried
- Vanilla extract

Oils and Fats

- Butter, grass-fed
- Extra-virgin olive oil

Nuts and Seeds

- Nuts or seeds of your choice within the plan
- Peanut butter
- Pepitas (hulled pumpkin seeds)
- Walnuts

Sweeteners

- Honey
- Maple syrup, pure
- Stevia
- Sugar, granulated and brown

Rice and Pasta

- Bread, gluten-free whole-grain
- Bread crumbs, gluten-free (read ingredients and make sure it doesn't contain powdered garlic or onion)
- Cornmeal
- Cornstarch
- Popcorn kernels
- Rice, brown
- Spaghetti, gluten-free
- Tortillas, corn

Canned

- Pumpkin
- Lentils

GERD-FRIENDLY INGREDIENT SUBSTITUTIONS

REMOVE	REPLACE
Full-fat mayonnaise	Fat-free mayonnaise or nonfat Greek yogurt
Premade broth	Homemade broth
Garlic powder/garlic salt	Basil, ground cumin, Dijon mustard, ground mustard, Italian seasoning
Lemon, lime, or orange juice	Lemon, lime, or orange zest
Chili powder	Ground cumin, ground coriander
Paprika	Ground cumin
Cayenne pepper	Ground cumin
Shortening/butter	Extra-virgin olive oil, small amount grass-fed butter
Ketchup	Anchovy fillets or paste, fish sauce, gluten-free soy sauce (tamari), toasted sesame oil
MSG	Salt, gluten-free soy sauce (tamari), fish sauce

continued ▶

REMOVE	REPLACE
Onion powder	Fresh or ground ginger, salt, ground cumin, ground coriander
Salad dressing	Salad dressing made with lactose-free nonfat Greek yogurt, low-fat milk, or nut milks and herbs
Canned tomatoes	Dijon mustard, gluten-free soy sauce (tamari), fish sauce, anchovy paste
Pepper	Oregano, Italian seasoning, ground cumin, thyme
Oil-packed tuna	Water-packed tuna
Barbecue sauce	Liquid smoke, fish sauce, gluten-free soy sauce (tamari), Dijon mustard

Love and Support Your Digestive System

Your digestive system is one of the most important systems in your body. It's the foundation for health. You may have heard the saying "you are what you eat," but I tell my patients and people who attend my workshops that the statement is not strictly true: In fact, you are what you digest and absorb. If this system is not working properly, all the money and time you spend on your meals will be wasted. Problems with digestion and gut inflammation are at the root of acid reflux, heartburn, and many other diseases.

Your digestive system is your body's largest barrier, protecting the rest of your cells and organs from any foreign invaders and substances such as chemicals, microbes, and microbe toxins. Think about this: Your digestive tract is made of a single layer of cells that is more fragile than your skin. If you cut or bruise your skin, you take care of it. But you can't see your gut, which is larger and more sensitive than your skin.

Having acid reflux symptoms, or any other digestive symptom, is your body's way of telling you that something is off, that something is not right and needs to be fixed. This is exactly what you were paying attention to when you decided to pick up this book. You may have ignored your body's message in the past (we can all be guilty of that), but now is the time to answer its call and start to heal yourself.

Recipe Labels

The recipes in part 2 are designed to fit within the STOP and HEAL plans. Some will also fit into the REINTRODUCE plan; however, you can add a bit of the foods you are reintroducing to any recipe if you wish. None are written specifically for the REINTRODUCE plan. Each recipe will have one or more labels. The following are descriptions of what you can expect of recipes with each label.

MEAL PLAN

These labels tell you if it is safe to consume these recipes in a particular meal plan:

- **STOP recipes:** These are designed for the 3-day STOP plan, which can help you soothe acid reflux quickly. The ingredients in these recipes have a pH of 6 or higher (a few may be in the 5 to 6 range, but these are limited), are low in fat, have small portion sizes, and omit ingredients that are likely to cause acid reflux such as chiles, bell peppers, onions, garlic, caffeine, chocolate, coffee, and alcohol. They also omit sugar except for honey or pure maple syrup.
- **HEAL recipes:** These are designed for the 4-week HEAL plan, which you will use as an elimination diet to allow your acid reflux to heal completely. These recipes omit chiles, onions, garlic, bell peppers, and foods that are high in FODMAPs. They are also low in fat and portion-controlled.
- **REINTRODUCE recipes:** These are the same as HEAL recipes. However, you can use these recipes to reintroduce foods one at a time, such as adding a small amount of tomato to a chili recipe. Look at the recipe tips at the end of each recipe for REINTRODUCE tips.

RECIPE EASE

These labels give you information about the ease of the recipes. All recipes have one or more of these labels.

- **5-Ingredient:** All recipes contain ten or fewer total ingredients, but these recipes contain five or fewer main ingredients. Salt, oil, and water are not included in the count.
- **30-Minute:** These recipes can be made from start to finish in 30 minutes or less, so they're great for busy weeknight meals.
- **One-Pan:** You can make the recipe in a single pan, minimizing cleanup time.
- **One-Pot:** You can make the entire recipe in a single pot, minimizing cleanup time.
- **Recipe Tips:** All of the recipes have a tip at the end. These tips offer ways to customize or boost flavor, or suggest ingredients you can add or subtract to fit into other plans. Be sure to check the tips to make sure you are preparing it properly for the meal plan you are following.

Part II

Recipes That Prevent Acid Reflux

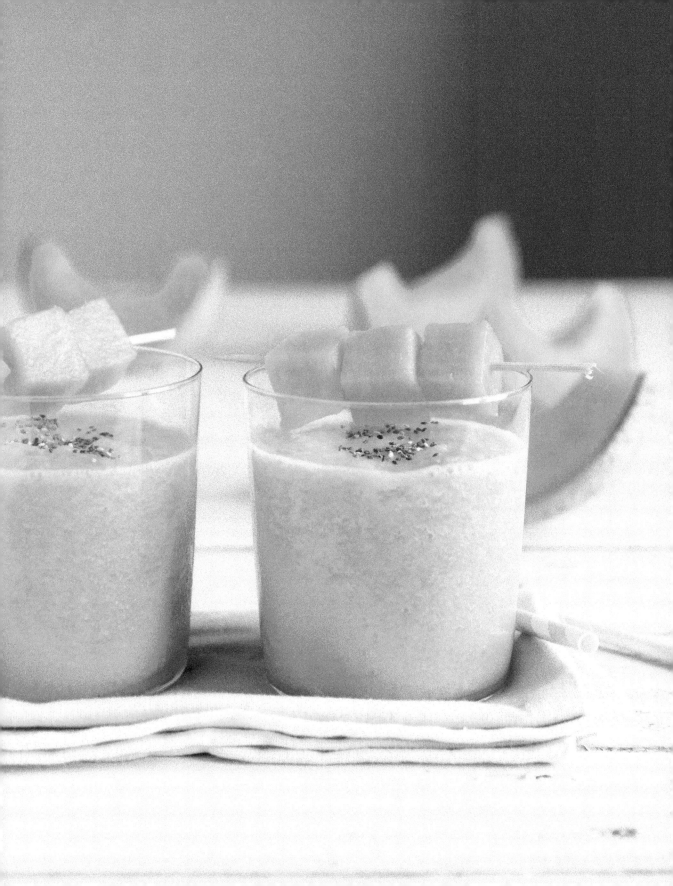

4

Breakfast and Brunch

Banana-Flax Smoothie 70

Sweet Melon Smoothie 71

Green Aloe Vera Smoothie 72

Chia Breakfast Pudding with Cantaloupe 73

Fruit and Yogurt Parfait 74

Apple Compote Smoothie 75

Maple-Ginger Oatmeal 76

Corn Porridge with Maple and Raisins 77

Raisin Cornmeal Pancakes 78

French Toast 79

Banana Pancakes 80

Sweet Potato Hash 81

Toads in a Hole 82

Turkey and Egg Breakfast Sandwich 83

Turkey Breakfast Sausage 84

Baked Avocado and Egg 85

Spinach Frittata 86

Salmon and Egg Scramble 87

Mushroom and Herb Omelet 88

Puffy Omelet 89

Sweet Melon Smoothie, page 71

Banana-Flax Smoothie

PREP TIME: 5 MINUTES

Smoothies are a quick way to start your day with a nutritious breakfast. Split the smoothie in half to keep from overfilling your belly. You can take the second half with you in a thermos for a mid-morning snack. SERVES 2

5-INGREDIENT
30-MINUTE
ONE-PAN

1 banana

1½ cups nondairy milk
(such as rice milk) or
lactose-free nonfat milk

2 tablespoons flaxseed

¼ teaspoon vanilla extract

¼ teaspoon
ground nutmeg

1 packet stevia (optional)

½ cup crushed ice

In a blender, combine all the ingredients and blend until smooth.

FLAVOR BOOST: Add ½ teaspoon ground ginger or grated fresh ginger to boost flavor and soothe flaring acid reflux. For REINTRODUCE, you can replace the banana with ½ cup chopped mango.

Serving size: 1½ cups Calories: 138; Protein: 3g; Total fat: 7g; Saturated fat: 1g; Carbohydrates: 18g; Fiber: 5g; Sodium: 130mg

Sweet Melon Smoothie

Melon is soothing to acid reflux, and it has a luscious, sweet flavor. Choose any melon except watermelon for this smoothie. To save even more time when you're in a hurry, you can purchase chopped melon from the produce section or salad bar of your local grocery store. SERVES 2

5-INGREDIENT

30-MINUTE

ONE-PAN

1½ cups chopped
   cantaloupe or
   other melon

1½ cups nondairy milk
   (such as rice milk) or
   lactose-free nonfat milk

½ cup lactose-free plain
   nonfat yogurt

¼ teaspoon ground
   fennel seed

1 packet stevia (optional)

½ cup crushed ice

In a blender, combine all the ingredients and blend until smooth.

SUBSTITUTION: For the STOP plan, you can substitute chopped papaya for the melon to change the flavor profile. For REINTRODUCE, you can substitute chopped papaya, chopped pineapple, or berries for the melon.

Serving size: 1½ cups Calories: 108; Protein: 5g; Total fat: 3g; Saturated fat: 1g; Carbohydrates: 16g; Fiber: 2g; Sodium: 188mg

STOP

HEAL

Green Aloe Vera Smoothie

PREP TIME: 5 MINUTES

This easy smoothie is packed with nutritious greens to give you a boost of vitamins, minerals, and other nutrients as you head out the door. Aloe vera is a soothing ingredient, so this is also a good smoothie to enjoy if you're noticing any pain. SERVES 2

5-INGREDIENT
30-MINUTE
ONE-PAN

1½ cups baby spinach

¼ cup fresh parsley

½ banana

1½ cups aloe vera

1 packet stevia (optional)

½ cup crushed ice

In a blender, combine all the ingredients and blend until smooth.

FLAVOR BOOST: Add ½ teaspoon ground cinnamon to add a sweet spiciness to this smoothie.

Serving size: 1½ cups Calories: 158; Protein: 3g; Total fat: <1g; Saturated fat: <1g; Carbohydrates: 39g; Fiber: 3g; Sodium: 23mg

Chia Breakfast Pudding with Cantaloupe

Make this pudding the night before to give the chia time to gel. Then in the morning you can get up, chop the fruit, and enjoy a quick and easy breakfast. The pudding without the added fruit will keep well in the refrigerator for up to 5 days. SERVES 4

5-INGREDIENT
ONE-PAN

2 cups lactose-free nonfat milk or nondairy milk (such as rice milk)

¼ cup honey

½ teaspoon vanilla extract

½ cup chia seeds

1 cup chopped cantaloupe

1. In a bowl, whisk together the milk, honey, and vanilla.

2. Stir in the chia seeds. Cover and refrigerate overnight (or for at least 4 hours).

3. Serve the cantaloupe spooned over the pudding.

SUBSTITUTION: To make this suitable for the HEAL or REINTRODUCE plan, replace the honey with pure maple syrup or 2 packets stevia. For REINTRODUCE, you can replace half of the cantaloupe with ½ cup berries or chopped pineapple.

Serving size: 1 cup Calories: 206; Protein: 7g; Total fat: 7g; Saturated fat: 1g; Carbohydrates: 34g; Fiber: 8g; Sodium: 81mg

STOP

REINTRODUCE

Fruit and Yogurt Parfait

PREP TIME: 10 MINUTES

Parfaits can be as easy or complex as you like. While this recipe calls for layering, it's purely a visual effect. If you're in a hurry, you can just put all the ingredients in a bowl. It won't be as pretty, but it will taste just as good. This will keep in the refrigerator for up to 3 days, but if you choose to refrigerate it for longer than a few hours, wait to add the pecans until just before you eat. SERVES 2

REINTRODUCE

5-INGREDIENT

30-MINUTE

2 cups lactose-free plain nonfat yogurt

3 tablespoons pure maple syrup

¼ teaspoon ground ginger

½ banana, peeled and sliced

¼ cup chopped pecans

1. In a small bowl, whisk together the yogurt, syrup, and ginger.

2. Spoon ½ cup of the yogurt mixture into each of two parfait glasses.

3. Top each with half of the banana slices.

4. Top each with another ½ cup yogurt mixture.

5. Sprinkle each with 2 tablespoons pecans.

SUBSTITUTION: To make this suitable for HEAL, replace the banana with cantaloupe balls. For REINTRODUCE, try substituting ½ cup chopped red apple for the banana.

Serving size: 1½ cups Calories: 354; Protein: 14g; Total fat: 14g; Saturated fat: 3g; Carbohydrates: 46g; Fiber: 2g; Sodium: 175mg

Apple Compote Smoothie

PREP TIME: 5 MINUTES (PLUS COOLING TIME); COOK TIME: 15 MINUTES

You'll need to use red apples here (such as Red Delicious), which are lower in acid than green apples. Allow the apple compote to cool completely before blending; you can make it up to 5 days ahead of time and refrigerate it. SERVES 2

5-INGREDIENT

1 red apple, peeled, cored, and chopped

2 tablespoons water

1 packet stevia

½ teaspoon ground cinnamon

1½ cups lactose-free nonfat milk

½ cup crushed ice

1. In a medium pot, combine the apple and water. Bring to a simmer over medium-high heat, stirring occasionally.

2. Reduce the heat to medium and cook until the apple is soft, about 10 minutes.

3. Stir in the stevia and cinnamon. Set aside to cool completely.

4. Combine the compote, milk, and ice in a blender and blend until smooth.

FLAVOR BOOST: For a different flavor profile, add 1 teaspoon grated orange zest and replace the cinnamon with ½ teaspoon ground cardamom.

Serving size: 2 cups Calories: 129; Protein: 8g; Total fat: 1g; Saturated fat: <1g; Carbohydrates: 24g; Fiber: 1g; Sodium: 109mg

Maple-Ginger Oatmeal

PREP TIME: 5 MINUTES; COOK TIME: 10 MINUTES

Oatmeal is moderately high in FODMAPs, so if you choose to consume this during the HEAL or REINTRODUCE plans (see Substitution), you'll want to limit your portion to ¼ cup. Since this makes a pretty small meal, consider having half a banana or ¼ cup lactose-free plain nonfat yogurt to round out your meal. SERVES 2

5-INGREDIENT
30-MINUTE
ONE-PAN

1½ cups water

Pinch salt

1 cup old-fashioned
   rolled oats

¼ cup pure maple syrup

½ teaspoon ground ginger

1. In a small pot, bring the water and salt to a boil over medium-high heat.

2. Stir in the oats, syrup, and ginger.

3. Reduce the heat to medium-low. Cook, stirring frequently, for 5 minutes.

SUBSTITUTION: To make this entirely friendly for all three plans, turn it into a breakfast quinoa. Increase water to 2 cups and substitute 1 cup quinoa for the oats. Cook, stirring, for 15 minutes. For REINTRODUCE, add ½ cup chopped red apples as you cook.

Serving size: ½ cup Calories: 258; Protein: 7g; Total fat: 3g; Saturated fat: <1g; Carbohydrates: 53g; Fiber: 4g; Sodium: 53mg

Corn Porridge with Maple and Raisins

PREP TIME: 5 MINUTES; COOK TIME: 15 MINUTES

Cornmeal makes a creamy breakfast porridge. If you like your hot cereal with a little milk, feel free to add up to ¼ cup of lactose-free nonfat milk to your porridge. Or top it with a dollop of lactose-free plain nonfat yogurt, which has a nice sourness to balance the sweetness of the corn, maple, and raisins. SERVES 2

5-INGREDIENT
30-MINUTE

¾ cup cornmeal

2¼ cups water, divided

Pinch salt

1 tablespoon pure
    maple syrup

½ teaspoon grated
    orange zest

Pinch ground nutmeg

3 tablespoons raisins

1. In a small bowl, whisk together the cornmeal and ¾ cup of water.

2. In a small pot, bring the remaining 1½ cups of water and the salt to a boil over medium-high heat.

3. Whisk in the cornmeal slurry. Cook, stirring, for 10 to 12 minutes, until thick.

4. Stir in the maple syrup, orange zest, nutmeg, and raisins. Serve hot.

SUBSTITUTION: For REINTRODUCE, omit the raisins. Instead, stir in ½ pear, peeled and chopped, just before serving.

Serving size: 1 cup Calories: 288; Protein: 6g; Total fat: 3g; Saturated fat: 1g; Carbohydrates: 60g; Fiber: 6g; Sodium: 53mg

Raisin Cornmeal Pancakes

PREP TIME: 5 MINUTES; COOK TIME: 15 MINUTES

These tender pancakes make a delicious breakfast. Top them with a little maple syrup or, if you are on the STOP plan, a squeeze of honey. You can find all-purpose gluten-free flour in many health food stores, online, or at grocery stores such as Whole Foods that have dedicated gluten-free sections. SERVES 4

HEAL
REINTRODUCE

30-MINUTE

1 cup lactose-free nonfat milk

2 tablespoons olive oil, plus more for the pan

1 tablespoon pure maple syrup

2 large eggs

1 cup cornmeal

¼ cup all-purpose gluten-free flour

1½ teaspoons baking powder

½ teaspoon ground cinnamon

Pinch salt

¼ cup raisins

1. In a small bowl, whisk together the milk, oil, syrup, and eggs.

2. In a medium bowl, whisk together the cornmeal, flour, baking powder, cinnamon, and salt.

3. Fold the wet ingredients into the dry ingredients until just mixed. There will be streaks of flour remaining in the batter.

4. Fold in the raisins.

5. Heat a nonstick skillet over medium-high heat. Brush with a little oil just to coat the pan.

6. Working in batches, ladle ¼ cup of batter for each pancake into the hot skillet. Cook until bubbles form, about 2 minutes. Flip and cook for an additional 2 minutes.

SUBSTITUTION: To make this suitable for STOP, replace the raisins with banana chips. If you are following REINTRODUCE, replace the raisins with ¼ cup blueberries.

Serving size: 2 pancakes Calories: 358; Protein: 10g; Total fat: 12g; Saturated fat: 2g; Carbohydrates: 53g; Fiber: 4g; Sodium: 95mg

French Toast

PREP TIME: 5 MINUTES; COOK TIME: 10 MINUTES

Use a gluten-free sandwich bread here, such as Udi's gluten-free sandwich bread, which you can find in the freezer section of most grocery stores. If you're a purist, top the French toast with a little maple syrup. Otherwise, try a tablespoon of peanut butter and half a sliced banana. SERVES 4

30-MINUTE

1½ cups lactose-free nonfat milk

2 large eggs, beaten

½ teaspoon vanilla extract

1 teaspoon grated orange zest

1 packet stevia

½ teaspoon ground nutmeg

Pinch salt

4 slices gluten-free sandwich bread

1 teaspoon unsalted grass-fed butter

1. In a small bowl, whisk together the milk, eggs, vanilla, orange zest, stevia, nutmeg, and salt.

2. Pour into a shallow dish. Soak the bread in the custard for 2 minutes, flipping once to coat.

3. Melt the butter in a nonstick skillet over medium-high heat.

4. Add the bread and cook for 2 to 3 minutes per side, until the custard sets and browns.

FLAVOR BOOST: Add ½ teaspoon ground cardamom to the custard and sprinkle each piece with 1 tablespoon confectioners' sugar before serving.

Serving size: 1 slice Calories: 148; Protein: 10g; Total fat: 5g; Saturated fat: 2g; Carbohydrates: 17g; Fiber: 2g; Sodium: 239mg

Banana Pancakes

PREP TIME: 5 MINUTES; COOK TIME: 10 MINUTES

These pancakes are so easy—they use just two ingredients and a tiny bit of butter. For best results, use a very ripe banana, like the type you'd use to make banana bread.

SERVES 2

5-INGREDIENT

30-MINUTE

1 ripe banana, peeled

2 large eggs, beaten

1 teaspoon unsalted grass-fed butter

1. In a small bowl, mash the banana.

2. Whisk in the eggs.

3. Melt the butter in a nonstick skillet over medium-high heat.

4. Scoop the banana mixture into the skillet to make four pancakes. Cook for about 1 minute per side.

FLAVOR BOOST: Top these pancakes with 1 tablespoon peanut butter for a tasty and fun breakfast.

Serving size: 2 pancakes Calories: 149; Protein: 7g; Total fat: 7g; Saturated fat: 3g; Carbohydrates: 16g; Fiber: 2g; Sodium: 71mg

Sweet Potato Hash

PREP TIME: 10 MINUTES; COOK TIME: 20 MINUTES

You can also make this hash with russet potatoes. Serve it topped with an egg prepared in any way for a full and flavorful meal. You can store and refrigerate this for up to 3 days and reheat it in the microwave, but it tastes best fresh from the stove top. SERVES 2

5-INGREDIENT

30-MINUTE

ONE-PAN

1 tablespoon olive oil

1 large sweet potato, peeled and cut into ½-inch cubes

½ teaspoon dried thyme

½ teaspoon sea salt

1. In a medium nonstick skillet over medium-high heat, heat the oil until it shimmers.

2. Add the sweet potato, thyme, and salt. Cook, stirring, for about 4 minutes, until the potatoes start to brown.

3. Lower the heat to medium. Cook, stirring occasionally, until the potatoes are deeply browned, about 15 minutes.

FLAVOR BOOST: Add ¼ teaspoon ground cumin in place of the thyme. Stir a bit of chopped fresh cilantro into the potatoes just before serving. Serve topped with 2 tablespoons lactose-free nonfat plain yogurt.

Serving size: ¼ cup Calories: 116; Protein: 1g; Total fat: 7g; Saturated fat: 1g; Carbohydrates: 13g; Fiber: 2g; Sodium: 617mg

Toads in a Hole

PREP TIME: 5 MINUTES; COOK TIME: 10 MINUTES

This simple breakfast is so satisfying. With half a banana on the side, you've got a satisfying and complete meal that will carry you through your morning with energy to spare. For best results, crack your eggs into a ramekin and slide them into the hole in the bread instead of cracking them directly into the bread. SERVES 2

5-INGREDIENT
30-MINUTE

2 pieces gluten-free
  sandwich bread, toasted
1 tablespoon olive oil
2 large eggs
Pinch sea salt

1. Cut out a hole large enough to hold an egg in the center of the toasted bread. Brush both sides of the toast with olive oil.

2. Heat a nonstick skillet over medium heat. Add the bread. Carefully (without breaking the yolks) crack one egg into a ramekin and then slide the egg into the hole in the toast. Repeat with the other egg. Season each with sea salt.

3. Cook until the eggs are set around the edges, 2 to 3 minutes.

4. Carefully flip the bread and eggs with a spatula and turn off the heat. Cook for about 1 minute more.

FLAVOR BOOST: Try a flavored sea salt, such as truffle salt (you can find it online) or smoked salt in place of the regular sea salt. It adds a wonderful pop of flavor.

Serving size: 1 piece Calories: 198; Protein: 9g; Total fat: 13g; Saturated fat: 3g; Carbohydrates: 12g; Fiber: 1g; Sodium: 225mg

Turkey and Egg Breakfast Sandwich

PREP TIME: 5 MINUTES; COOK TIME: 10 MINUTES

Breakfast sandwiches are perfect for meals on the run. They come together quickly, and they're portable. If you don't wish to cut the sandwich in half to make two servings, you can also make it open-faced, with the egg and turkey divided between two pieces of bread. SERVES 2

5-INGREDIENT
30-MINUTE
ONE-PAN

1 tablespoon olive oil

3 ounces plain deli turkey, chopped

3 large eggs, beaten

½ teaspoon sea salt

2 pieces gluten-free sandwich bread, toasted

1. In a medium nonstick skillet, heat the olive oil over medium-high heat until it shimmers.

2. Add the turkey and cook, stirring, until it starts to crisp, about 3 minutes. Lower the heat to medium.

3. Add the eggs and salt. Cook, stirring to scramble, until the eggs are set, 2 to 3 minutes.

4. Spoon the turkey and eggs onto one piece of toast. Top with the other piece. Cut in half to serve.

SUBSTITUTION: Once you add honey in REINTRODUCE, you may try honey-flavored varieties of deli turkey.

Serving size: ½ sandwich Calories: 280; Protein: 18g; Total fat: 16g; Saturated fat: 4g; Carbohydrates: 16g; Fiber: 1g; Sodium: 1321mg

Turkey Breakfast Sausage

PREP TIME: 5 MINUTES; COOK TIME: 10 MINUTES

Most sausages contain garlic, which can wreak havoc on acid reflux. But when you make your own, you control the ingredients and you get to have a delicious, super easy, and fast breakfast treat. These patties keep well once they've been cooked (3 days in the refrigerator or up to 3 months in the freezer), and you can reheat them in the microwave. SERVES 4

5-INGREDIENT
30-MINUTE

12 ounces ground turkey breast

1 tablespoon dried sage

½ teaspoon dried marjoram

½ teaspoon ground fennel seed

½ teaspoon sea salt

1 teaspoon unsalted grass-fed butter

1. In a bowl, combine the ground turkey, sage, marjoram, fennel, and salt. Form into 8 patties.

2. Melt the butter in a nonstick skillet over medium-high heat.

3. Add the sausage patties and cook until browned, about 4 minutes per side.

FLAVOR BOOST: Looking for a different flavor profile? Trade the sage, marjoram, and fennel for 1 tablespoon dried oregano, 1 teaspoon ground cumin, and ½ teaspoon ground coriander.

Serving size: 2 (1½-ounce) patties Calories: 135; Protein: 15g; Total fat: 8g; Saturated fat: 3g; Carbohydrates: <1g; Fiber: <1g; Sodium: 370mg

Baked Avocado and Egg

PREP TIME: 10 MINUTES; COOK TIME: 20 MINUTES

This simple yet flavorful breakfast has gained in popularity recently. Baking an avocado increases its grassy, green flavors and firms the texture a bit. These don't keep, so plan on making only as many as you can serve or eat in the moment. If you're cooking just for yourself, halve the recipe and refrigerate the other avocado half for another time. SERVES 2

5-INGREDIENT
30-MINUTE
ONE-PAN

1 avocado, halved
  lengthwise and pitted

2 large eggs

½ teaspoon sea salt

1. Preheat the oven to 450°F.

2. Place the avocado halves cut-side up on a rimmed baking sheet. Spoon out about half of the avocado flesh (refrigerate it for later in a tightly sealed container) from the center to make room for the eggs.

3. Carefully crack an egg into the center of each avocado half.

4. Bake until the eggs are set, 15 to 20 minutes.

5. Season with the salt.

SUBSTITUTION: If you're watching FODMAPs in the HEAL plan, you can have ⅛ avocado. So while you can't bake an egg in an avocado, you can make a version of this by scrambling or frying the egg and topping with ⅛ avocado, chopped.

Serving size: ½ avocado, 1 egg Calories: 185; Protein: 8g; Total fat: 15g; Saturated fat: 3g; Carbohydrates: 6g; Fiber: 5g; Sodium: 657mg

STOP

REINTRODUCE

Spinach Frittata

PREP TIME: 10 MINUTES; COOK TIME: 10 MINUTES

You'll need an oven-safe pan for this, one with handles that won't melt under the broiler. Cast iron works well here, as do stainless steel and similar surfaces. Cut the frittata in half to serve. SERVES 2

5-INGREDIENT
30-MINUTE

1 tablespoon olive oil

2 cups baby spinach

4 large eggs

¼ cup lactose-free
nonfat milk

½ teaspoon sea salt

1. Preheat the broiler on high.

2. In a medium oven-safe skillet, heat the oil over medium-high heat until it shimmers.

3. Add the spinach and cook, stirring, until it is wilted, about 3 minutes.

4. In a small bowl, whisk together the eggs, milk, and salt.

5. Pour the egg mixture carefully over the spinach. Lower the heat to medium.

6. Cook until the eggs begin to set around the edges, about 2 minutes.

7. Using a spatula, carefully pull the set eggs away from the sides of the skillet. Tilt the skillet to distribute the uncooked egg into the spaces you've made. Cook until the eggs set around the edges again, 2 to 3 minutes more.

8. Transfer the skillet to the broiler. Broil until set on top, 2 to 3 minutes.

9. Cut into wedges and serve.

FLAVOR BOOST: Sprinkle the top of the frittata with 1½ ounces grated Parmesan cheese just before you put it under the broiler.

SUBSTITUTION: For REINTRODUCE, sauté ½ cup sliced mushrooms along with the spinach.

Serving size: ½ frittata Calories: 220; Protein: 14g; Total fat: 17g; Saturated fat: 4g; Carbohydrates: 3g; Fiber: 1g; Sodium: 761mg

Salmon and Egg Scramble

When you buy the smoked salmon, read the ingredients label carefully to make sure it hasn't been cured with honey or seasoned with any added ingredients such as garlic or onion. If you can't find smoked salmon that meet these criteria, you can use canned salmon that you have drained, rinsed, and patted dry with a paper towel. SERVES 2

5-INGREDIENT
30-MINUTE
ONE-PAN

1 tablespoon olive oil

3 ounces smoked
   salmon, flaked

4 large eggs, beaten

1 teaspoon dried tarragon

½ teaspoon sea salt

1. In a large nonstick skillet, heat the oil over medium-high heat until it shimmers.

2. Add the salmon, eggs, tarragon, and salt. Cook, stirring occasionally to scramble, until the eggs set, about 4 minutes.

FLAVOR BOOST: If you're on HEAL or REINTRODUCE, you can create an avocado lemon crema to top the scramble. To make it, combine ⅛ avocado, 2 tablespoons lactose-free nonfat plain yogurt, a pinch of sea salt, and ½ teaspoon grated lemon zest in a blender. Blend until smooth. Dollop a tablespoon or two on top of your eggs.

Serving size: about ½ cup Calories: 253; Protein: 20g; Total fat: 19g; Saturated fat: 4g; Carbohydrates: 1g; Fiber: 0g; Sodium: 1051mg

STOP

HEAL

REINTRODUCE

Mushroom and Herb Omelet

PREP TIME: 5 MINUTES; COOK TIME: 10 MINUTES

Mushrooms add a distinctly earthy flavor to this omelet, and thyme is the perfect accompaniment for the mushrooms. This omelet will store and reheat well. Save it, tightly sealed, in the refrigerator for up to 3 days and reheat on high in the microwave for 1 to 1½ minutes. SERVES 2

5-INGREDIENT
30-MINUTE
ONE-PAN

1 tablespoon olive oil

1 cup sliced mushrooms

½ teaspoon dried thyme

½ teaspoon sea salt

4 large eggs, beaten

1. In a medium nonstick pan, heat the oil over medium-high heat until it shimmers. Add the mushrooms, thyme, and salt. Cook, stirring occasionally, until brown, about 5 minutes.

2. Lower the heat to medium. Spread the mushrooms in an even layer on the bottom of the pan. Carefully pour the eggs over the top.

3. Cook undisturbed until the eggs set on the edges, about 3 minutes. Using a spatula, carefully pull the eggs away from the edges of the pan. Tilt the pan to allow the uncooked eggs to run into the spaces you made. Cook until the eggs set again, about 3 minutes more.

4. Carefully fold the omelet in half. Slide onto a platter and cut in half to serve.

FLAVOR BOOST: Add ¼ cup grated Cheddar cheese before you fold the omelet. Spread it in a single layer, fold the omelet, turn off the heat, and allow the cheese to melt before serving.

Serving size: ½ omelet Calories: 211; Protein: 14g; Total fat: 17g; Saturated fat: 4g; Carbohydrates: 2g; Fiber: <1g; Sodium: 723mg

Puffy Omelet

PREP TIME: 10 MINUTES; COOK TIME: 10 MINUTES

This omelet seems fancy, but it's really simple and has only two ingredients: eggs and salt (plus oil for the pan). The result is super fluffy, light, and delicious. If you want, you can top it with sautéed veggies or serve it with a side of Sweet Potato Hash (page 81). SERVES 2

5-INGREDIENT
30-MINUTE

2 large eggs, separated
¼ teaspoon sea salt
1 teaspoon olive oil

1. In a medium bowl, beat the egg whites with an egg-beater on high speed until they form stiff peaks, about 5 minutes.

2. In a small bowl, whisk the egg yolks with the salt until well combined.

3. Fold the egg whites into the egg yolks until combined, being careful not to flatten the fluffy whites.

4. Heat the oil in a small nonstick pan over medium-high heat until it shimmers.

5. Lower the heat to medium. Pour the egg mixture into the pan, using a rubber spatula to scrape the eggs from the sides of the bowl. Smooth the surface of the eggs in the pan with the spatula.

6. Cook until the eggs set, 5 to 6 minutes. Carefully fold the omelet in half, then slide it onto a plate.

FLAVOR BOOST: Sprinkle 2 tablespoons grated Asiago or Parmesan cheese in the center of the omelet before folding it.

Serving size: ½ omelet Calories: 91; Protein: 6g; Total fat: 7g; Saturated fat: 2g; Carbohydrates: 0g; Fiber: 0g; Sodium: 361mg

STOP

HEAL

REINTRODUCE

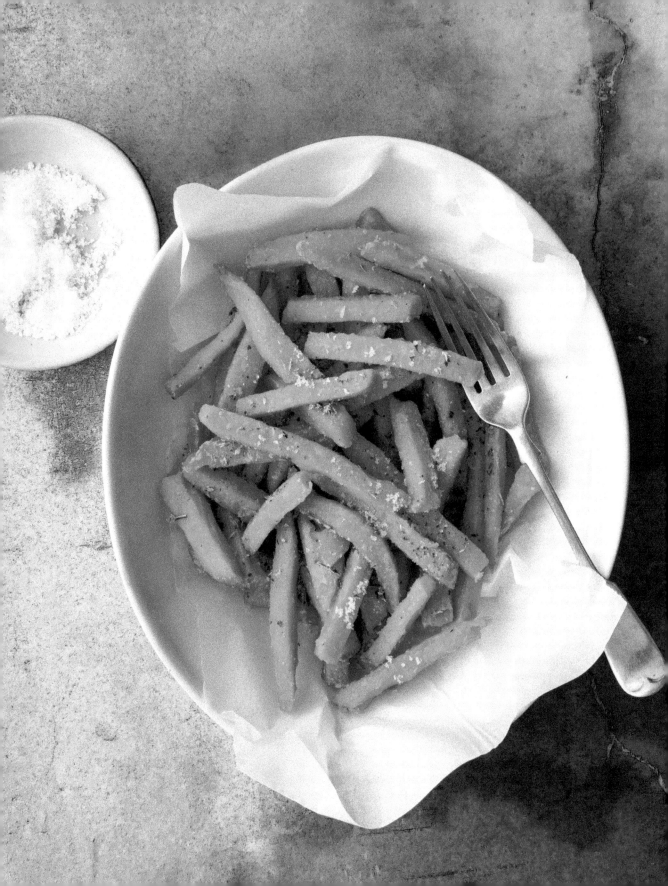

5

Appetizers and Sides

Spinach and Dill Dip 92

Zucchini Hummus 93

Zucchini and Salmon Canapés 94

Olive Tapenade 95

Sweet Potato French Fries 96

Artichoke Purée 97

Green Beans Amandine 98

Roasted Asparagus with
   Goat Cheese 99

Creamed Spinach 100

Mashed Potatoes 101

Quinoa Pilaf 102

Roasted Honey-Ginger Carrots 103

Chopped Kale Salad 104

Quick Pasta Salad 106

Sweet Potato French Fries, page 96

Spinach and Dill Dip

PREP TIME: 5 MINUTES (PLUS COOLING TIME); COOK TIME: 5 MINUTES

This bright, fresh dip is delicious with gluten-free crackers or carrot sticks. It makes a great snack and, in larger portions, a tasty appetizer. If you prefer a smoother dip, you can combine the cooled spinach mixture with the yogurt and dill in a blender or food processor and blend until smooth. It will keep in the refrigerator for 3 days. SERVES 4

5-INGREDIENT
30-MINUTE

1 tablespoon olive oil

2 cups baby spinach

**½ teaspoon grated
lemon zest**

¼ teaspoon sea salt

**1 cup lactose-free nonfat
plain yogurt**

**2 tablespoons chopped
fresh dill**

1. In a large nonstick skillet, heat the olive oil over medium-high heat until it shimmers.

2. Add the spinach, lemon zest, and sea salt. Cook, stirring, until the spinach wilts, 2 to 3 minutes. Remove from the heat and allow the spinach to cool.

3. In a small bowl, combine the cooled spinach, yogurt, and dill, stirring to combine.

SUBSTITUTION: To make this dairy-free, you can replace the yogurt with 1 cup crumbled tofu.

Serving size: ¼ cup Calories: 68; Protein: 4g; Total fat: 4g; Saturated fat: 1g; Carbohydrates: 5g; Fiber: 0g; Sodium: 205mg

Zucchini Hummus

PREP TIME: 5 MINUTES

Hummus can aggravate GERD because of its garlic content and the FODMAPs in chick-peas. This version replaces the chickpeas and garlic with zucchini and herbs but doesn't lose any flavor in the translation. Try it with gluten-free crackers, or carrots for dipping.

SERVES 4

5-INGREDIENT

30-MINUTE

ONE-PAN

1 medium
  zucchini, chopped

1 tablespoon olive oil

1 tablespoon tahini

1 teaspoon chopped
  fresh dill

½ teaspoon grated
  lemon zest

½ teaspoon sea salt

In a blender or food processor, combine all the ingredients. Blend until smooth.

FLAVOR BOOST: For REINTRODUCE, add ½ garlic clove, minced.

Serving size: ¼ cup Calories: 53; Protein: 1g; Total fat: 5g; Saturated fat: <1g; Carbohydrates: 1g; Fiber: 0g; Sodium: 295mg

Zucchini and Salmon Canapés

PREP TIME: 15 MINUTES

These make great snacks or, if you double or triple the recipe, a tasty appetizer for a crowd. Canned salmon gets a boost in flavor here from a fresh herb and orange zest, making it an appetizing dish. You can make the salmon topping ahead and refrigerate it for up to 3 days before putting it on the zucchini rounds. SERVES 4

5-INGREDIENT
30-MINUTE
ONE-PAN

4 ounces canned salmon,
  drained, rinsed,
  and flaked

¼ cup lactose-free nonfat
  plain yogurt

1 teaspoon grated
  orange zest

1 teaspoon chopped fresh
  tarragon

½ teaspoon sea salt

1 medium zucchini, cut
  into 12 rounds

1. In a small bowl, combine the salmon, yogurt, orange zest, tarragon, and salt.

2. Spoon onto the zucchini rounds.

SUBSTITUTION: You can substitute an equal amount of canned water-packed tuna for the salmon.

Serving size: 3 canapés Calories: 53; Protein: 7g; Total fat: 2g; Saturated fat: 1g; Carbohydrates: 1g; Fiber: 0g; Sodium: 323mg

Olive Tapenade

PREP TIME: 15 MINUTES

Spread olive tapenade on gluten-free toast or crackers for a tasty snack or appetizer. The tapenade keeps well, and it gets even better if it sits in the refrigerator overnight, allowing the flavors to blend. SERVES 4

5-INGREDIENT

30-MINUTE

ONE-PAN

½ cup pitted chopped black olives

½ anchovy fillet, finely chopped

1 tablespoon olive oil

2 tablespoons chopped fresh basil

½ teaspoon lemon zest

In a small bowl, mix all the ingredients until well combined.

FLAVOR BOOST: For REINTRODUCE, add ½ garlic clove, minced.

Serving size: 2 tablespoons Calories: 51; Protein: 0g; Total fat: 5g; Saturated fat: 1g; Carbohydrates: 1g; Fiber: 1g; Sodium: 165mg

STOP

HEAL

REINTRODUCE

Sweet Potato French Fries

PREP TIME: 10 MINUTES COOK TIME: 20 MINUTES

Sweet potatoes do have FODMAPs, but about half a small sweet potato (about ½ cup sweet potato fries) falls below the threshold for FODMAPs. However, if you find you are sensitive to sweet potatoes, you can use regular white potatoes to make these tasty fries.
SERVES 2

5-INGREDIENT
30-MINUTE

1 sweet potato, peeled and cut into ¼-inch matchsticks

1 teaspoon ground cumin

½ teaspoon sea salt

1 tablespoon olive oil

1. Preheat the oven to 450°F.

2. In a bowl, toss together the sweet potato sticks, cumin, salt, and olive oil.

3. Spread in a single layer on a rimmed baking sheet.

4. Bake, turning once with a spatula, until the fries are browned and tender, about 20 minutes.

SUBSTITUTION: If you want to make this with white potatoes, use one large russet potato. Omit the cumin.

Serving size: ½ cup Calories: 115; Protein: 1g; Total fat: 7g; Saturated fat: 1g; Carbohydrates: 14g; Fiber: 2g; Sodium: 619mg

Artichoke Purée

PREP TIME: 10 MINUTES COOK TIME: 5 MINUTES

This super quick purée is easy and delicious. It has a consistency similar to mashed potatoes, with the earthy and slightly sweet flavor of artichokes. If you are on the HEAL or REINTRODUCE plan, you can have about 2 tablespoons (½ serving) of this, but more might cause issues. Store in the refrigerator for up to 3 days and reheat to serve. SERVES 4

5-INGREDIENT

30-MINUTE

1 (14-ounce) can artichoke bottoms, drained

½ cup lactose-free nonfat milk or nondairy milk (such as rice milk)

1 tablespoon unsalted grass-fed butter

½ teaspoon sea salt

1. In a small saucepan, combine all the ingredients. Cook over medium-high heat, stirring occasionally, until warm, about 5 minutes.

2. Transfer to a blender or food processor and blend until smooth.

FLAVOR BOOST: Add ¼ cup grated Parmesan cheese to the blender or food processor before puréeing.

Serving size: ¼ cup Calories: 134; Protein: 4g; Total fat: 10g; Saturated fat: 2g; Carbohydrates: 12g; Fiber: 4g; Sodium: 694mg

STOP

Green Beans Amandine

PREP TIME: 10 MINUTES; COOK TIME: 15 MINUTES

Green beans with almonds is a perennial favorite side dish. To prepare the beans, trim the fibrous ends and then cut them in half. You can find slivered almonds in the baking aisle of most grocery stores. SERVES 2

5-INGREDIENT

30-MINUTE

¼ cup slivered almonds

24 green beans, trimmed and halved

1 tablespoon olive oil

½ teaspoon grated lemon zest

½ teaspoon sea salt

1. Preheat the oven to 350°F.

2. Spread the almonds in a single layer on a rimmed baking sheet and bake until toasted, about 5 minutes.

3. Fill a large pot halfway with water and bring to a boil over high heat. Add the beans and cook, covered, until tender, about 4 minutes. Drain.

4. Toss the beans with the toasted almonds, olive oil, lemon zest, and sea salt.

FLAVOR BOOST: Replace the almonds with an equal amount of pine nuts and omit the toasting step. Add 2 tablespoons grated Parmesan cheese when you toss all the ingredients together.

Serving size: ½ batch Calories: 185; Protein: 5g; Total fat: 16g; Saturated fat: 2g; Carbohydrates: 8g; Fiber: 4g; Sodium: 591mg

Roasted Asparagus with Goat Cheese

PREP TIME: 5 MINUTES; COOK TIME: 15 MINUTES

Just a sprinkle of goat cheese adds brightness to roasted asparagus. To prepare asparagus, snap off the woody ends by holding the spear in the middle and bending it. The spear will snap naturally in the right spot. Discard the ends. SERVES 2

5-INGREDIENT
30-MINUTE
ONE-PAN

10 asparagus spears

1 tablespoon olive oil

½ teaspoon sea salt

2 tablespoons crumbled
   goat cheese

½ teaspoon grated
   lemon zest

1. Preheat the oven to 425°F.

2. On a rimmed baking sheet, toss the asparagus with the olive oil and sea salt. Bake for 15 minutes, or until tender.

3. Sprinkle with the goat cheese and lemon zest before serving.

FLAVOR BOOST: Toast ¼ cup walnut pieces in a 350°F oven for 5 minutes and sprinkle over the asparagus for a toasty flavor and a nice crunch.

Serving size: ½ batch Calories: 94; Protein: 3g; Total fat: 8g; Saturated fat: 2g; Carbohydrates: 3g; Fiber: 2g; Sodium: 609mg

STOP

REINTRODUCE

Creamed Spinach

PREP TIME: 5 MINUTES; COOK TIME: 10 MINUTES

This creamy spinach is a tasty, comfort-food side that goes well with any meat or poultry main dish. A pinch of nutmeg brings out the best flavors in the spinach. It doesn't keep well, so plan on making this and serving it right away. SERVES 2

5-INGREDIENT
30-MINUTE

1 tablespoon olive oil

1 bunch spinach, stemmed
  and chopped

½ teaspoon sea salt

Pinch ground nutmeg

½ cup lactose-free
  nonfat milk

1 teaspoon cornstarch

1. In a large pot, heat the olive oil over medium-high heat until it shimmers. Add the spinach, salt, and nutmeg. Cook until the spinach is wilted, about 3 minutes.

2. In a small bowl, whisk together the milk and cornstarch. Add to the spinach. Cook, stirring, until the milk thickens, about 1 minute.

SUBSTITUTION: This also works well with other greens, such as kale, collards, or Swiss chard. Cooking these greens may take longer—5 to 7 minutes.

Serving size: ½ cup Calories: 135; Protein: 7g; Total fat: 8g; Saturated fat: 1g; Carbohydrates: 13g; Fiber: 4g; Sodium: 748mg

Mashed Potatoes

PREP TIME: 10 MINUTES; COOK TIME: 15 MINUTES

Mashed potatoes keep and reheat well. Store them tightly sealed in the refrigerator for up to 4 days, and reheat them in the microwave or add a bit more lactose-free milk and reheat them on the stove top. This is a classic accompaniment for meat or chicken.

SERVES 4

5-INGREDIENT
30-MINUTE
ONE-PAN

2 russet potatoes,
   peeled and cut into
   ½-inch cubes

½ cup lactose-free
   nonfat milk

2 tablespoons unsalted
   grass-fed butter, at room
   temperature

½ teaspoon sea salt

1. Put the potatoes in a large pot and cover with plenty of water. Cover and cook over high heat until the potatoes are soft, about 15 minutes. Drain the potatoes and return them to the pot.

2. Add the milk, butter, and salt. Mash with a potato masher until smooth. Taste for seasoning and add more salt if necessary.

SUBSTITUTION: You can also use this recipe to make smashed potatoes. Replace the russet potatoes with 4 unpeeled red potatoes, cut into ½-inch cubes. The skins will give extra texture to the potatoes.

Serving size: ½ cup Calories: 136; Protein: 3g; Total fat: 6g; Saturated fat: 4g; Carbohydrates: 21g; Fiber: 1g; Sodium: 313mg

Quinoa Pilaf

PREP TIME: 10 MINUTES; COOK TIME: 20 MINUTES

Quinoa has a toothsome bite that makes it a great grain side dish. This pilaf adds raisins for sweetness and pine nuts for a little extra crunch. It keeps and reheats well. You can refrigerate it for up to 4 days and reheat it in the microwave. SERVES 4

30-MINUTE
ONE-PAN

1 tablespoon olive oil

1 carrot, peeled
and chopped

½ cup quinoa, rinsed

1 cup Simple Vegetable
Broth (page 108)

¼ cup pine nuts

2 tablespoons raisins

2 tablespoons chopped
fresh parsley

½ teaspoon sea salt

1. In a medium pot, heat the oil over medium-high heat until it shimmers. Add the carrot and cook, stirring occasionally, until it starts to brown, about 5 minutes.

2. Add the quinoa and vegetable broth. Reduce to a simmer, cover, and cook until the quinoa is soft, about 15 minutes.

3. Add the pine nuts, raisins, parsley, and salt just before serving.

SUBSTITUTION: For STOP, omit the raisins.

Serving size: ½ cup Calories: 171; Protein: 4g; Total fat: 8g; Saturated fat: 1g; Carbohydrates: 23g; Fiber: 3g; Sodium: 369mg

Roasted Honey-Ginger Carrots

PREP TIME: 5 MINUTES; COOK TIME 20 MINUTES

Roasting carrots brings out their sweet, earthy flavors, and ginger and honey are the perfect complements to those flavors. Although it takes about 20 minutes to roast the carrots, the prep time is minimal, so it's a great dish for weeknights. SERVES 2

5-INGREDIENT

30-MINUTE

4 large carrots, peeled and cut lengthwise into quarters

2 tablespoons honey

1 tablespoon olive oil

1 teaspoon grated fresh ginger

½ teaspoon salt

1. Preheat the oven to 425°F.

2. Put the carrots in a single layer on a rimmed baking sheet.

3. In a small bowl, whisk together the honey, olive oil, ginger, and salt.

4. Drizzle over the carrots, turning to coat.

5. Bake until the carrots are tender, about 20 minutes.

SUBSTITUTION: To make this work for HEAL, replace the honey with 2 tablespoons pure maple syrup.

Serving size: 2 carrots Calories: 186; Protein: 1g; Total fat: 7g; Saturated fat: 1g; Carbohydrates: 32g; Fiber: 4g; Sodium: 682mg

Chopped Kale Salad

PREP TIME: 15 MINUTES

A crunchy kale salad adds a great textural element to any meal. This one has a creamy dressing with fresh herbs and orange zest that makes it taste like a delicious slaw. Most of the prep time comes in the form of chopping veggies. SERVES 2

HEAL

REINTRODUCE

30-MINUTE

2 cups stemmed and
   chopped kale

3 radishes, chopped

1 carrot, peeled
   and chopped

¼ cup lactose-free nonfat
   plain yogurt

1 teaspoon Dijon mustard

1 teaspoon chopped
   fresh thyme

1 teaspoon chopped
   fresh dill

½ teaspoon grated
   orange zest

½ teaspoon sea salt

1. In a large bowl, toss together the kale, radishes, and carrot.

2. In a small bowl, whisk together the yogurt, mustard, thyme, dill, orange zest, and sea salt.

3. Toss the dressing with the salad to serve.

SUBSTITUTION: For STOP, omit the mustard and replace the yogurt with ¼ cup crumbled tofu and 2 tablespoons lactose-free nonfat milk. Make the dressing in a blender instead of whisking it in a bowl.

Serving size: 1 cup Calories: 73; Protein: 4g; Total fat: <1g; Saturated fat: <1g; Carbohydrates: 13g; Fiber: 3g; Sodium: 687mg

Quick Pasta Salad

PREP TIME: 15 MINUTES

Pasta salad always makes a tasty side dish. This one uses the Creamy Herbed Dressing on page 200. You can make it the night before and refrigerate it. Serve it chilled. SERVES 4

30-MINUTE
ONE-PAN

2 cups cooked gluten-free
elbow macaroni

1 cup baby spinach

¼ cup canned chickpeas

¼ cup sliced black olives

¼ cup chopped fresh basil

1 recipe Creamy Herbed
Dressing (page 200)

1. In a large bowl, toss together the macaroni, spinach, chickpeas, olives, and basil.

2. Toss with the dressing.

SUBSTITUTION: For REINTRODUCE, add ¼ cup canned artichoke hearts, cut into quarters.

Serving size: 1 cup Calories: 152; Protein: 7g; Total fat: 2g; Saturated fat: <1g; Carbohydrates: 27g; Fiber: 4g; Sodium: 222mg

STOP

HEAL

REINTRODUCE

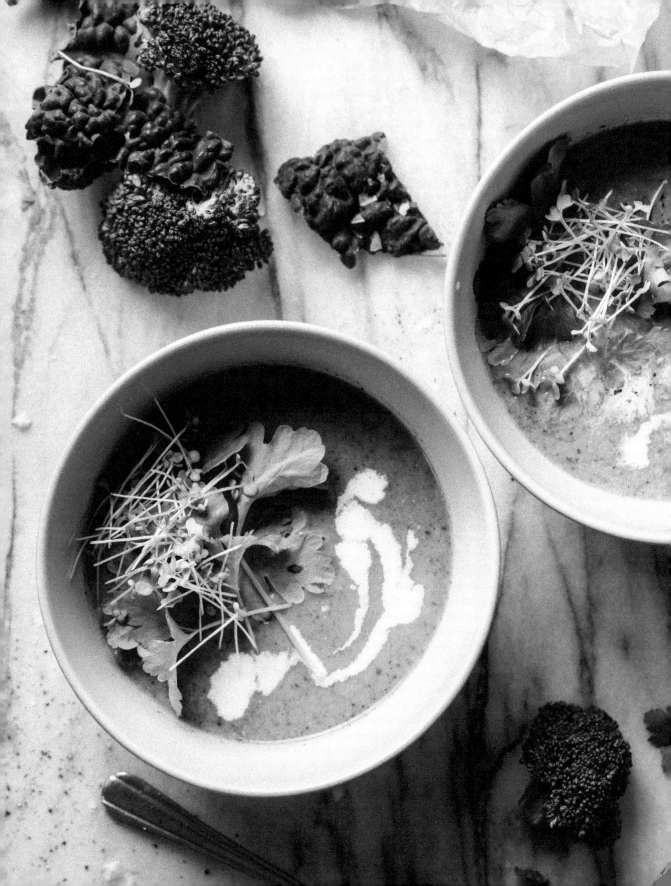

6

Vegetarian and Vegan

Simple Vegetable Broth 108

Cooling Cucumber Soup 109

Miso Soup with Tofu and Greens 110

Italian Vegetable Soup 111

Creamy Pumpkin Soup 112

Cream of Broccoli Soup 113

Sweet Potato and Corn Stew 114

Broccoli and Cheese Baked Potato 115

Lentil Tacos 116

Pasta with Walnut Pesto 117

Zucchini and Carrot Frittata 118

Zucchini Ribbons with
Parmesan Cream Sauce 119

Asian Veggie and Tofu Stir-Fry 120

Soba Noodles with
Peanut Butter Sauce 121

Brown Rice and Peanut
Lettuce Wraps 122

Vegetable and Tofu Fried Rice 123

Butternut Risotto 124

Brown Rice and Tofu with Kale 125

Seasoned Tofu with Chimichurri 126

Grilled Eggplant Burgers 127

Pesto Grilled Cheese 128

Fried Egg Sandwich 129

Cream of Broccoli Soup, page 113

Simple Vegetable Broth

PREP TIME: 10 MINUTES; COOK TIME: 2 HOURS

Simmering this broth takes time, but it's passive time. You can also make it in the slow cooker (just go for 8 hours on low instead of 2). Store the broth in one-cup servings in your freezer for up to a year, and you can just thaw what you need as you need it. SERVES 8

5-INGREDIENT
ONE-PAN

2 carrots, peeled and
   roughly chopped

1 leek, green part only,
   roughly chopped and
   washed (see headnote,
   page 110)

1 celery stalk,
   roughly chopped

1 fennel bulb,
   roughly chopped

9 cups water

1. In a large pot, combine all the ingredients.

2. Bring to a simmer over medium-high heat, then lower the heat to low and simmer for 2 hours.

3. Strain the vegetables from the broth and store the broth until you're ready to use it.

FLAVOR BOOST: For an Asian-flavored vegetable broth, add 2 whole star anise and 2 pieces peeled fresh ginger (about 1 inch each) to the broth to simmer as you cook it. You can also add herbs to the broth, such as a sprig of thyme or rosemary.

SUBSTITUTION: For REINTRODUCE, replace the leek with ½ small onion, roughly chopped.

Serving size: 1 cup Calories: 10; Protein: 0g; Total fat: 0g; Saturated fat: 0g; Carbohydrates: 3g; Fiber: 0g; Sodium: 20mg

Cooling Cucumber Soup

PREP TIME: 10 MINUTES (PLUS COOLING TIME);

Chilled soups are lovely on hot days. While this has no cooking time, you will need to chill it for a few hours so it is nice and cold when you serve it. Serve it as an attractive lunch dish or as the starter for a summer dinner. SERVES 4

4 medium cucumbers, roughly chopped

½ avocado, peeled, pitted, and roughly chopped

1 cup baby spinach, finely chopped

¼ cup chopped, fresh cilantro

1 teaspoon grated ginger root

Zest of 1 lime

½ teaspoon sea salt

3 cups Simple Vegetable Broth (page 108)

½ cup of lactose-free plain nonfat yogurt

2 tablespoons extra-virgin olive oil

Baby spinach leaves (optional, for garnish)

1. In a blender or food processor, combine the cucumbers, avocado, spinach, cilantro, ginger, lime zest, salt, vegetable broth, yogurt, and olive oil. Blend until smooth.

2. Chill for at least two hours.

3. Garnish with spinach leaves just prior to serving (if using).

SUBSTITUTION TIP: For REINTRODUCE, add 1 finely minced garlic clove to the soup as you puree it.

Serving size: About 2 cups Calories: 183; Protein: 4g; Total fat: 13g; Saturated Fat: 3g; Carbohydrates: 16g; Fiber: 4g; Sodium: 265mg

STOP

HEAL

REINTRODUCE

Miso Soup with Tofu and Greens

PREP TIME: 10 MINUTES; COOK TIME: 15 MINUTES

Miso adds a deep savory taste known as umami to this soup. While this recipe calls for spinach, you can substitute any greens, such as collards, kale, or Swiss chard. Be careful with the leek, as it can hold a lot of dirt. Cut the leek into pieces and put them in a bowl of water. Swish them around and allow the dirt to settle to the bottom. Empty the water and repeat the process until no more dirt settles at the bottom of the bowl. SERVES 4

5-INGREDIENT
30-MINUTE

1 tablespoon olive oil

1 leek, green part only, chopped and washed (see headnote)

3 ounces extra-firm tofu, cut into ¼-inch cubes

7 cups Simple Vegetable Broth (page 108), divided

3 cups baby spinach

2 tablespoons miso paste

1. In a large nonstick pot, heat the olive oil over medium-high heat until it shimmers.

2. Add the leek and tofu and cook, stirring occasionally, until the leek is soft, about 5 minutes.

3. Add 6 cups of broth. Bring to a simmer and lower the heat to medium.

4. Add the spinach. Cook for 3 minutes.

5. In a small bowl, whisk together the remaining 1 cup of broth and the miso paste. Stir into the hot soup. Cook for 30 seconds more, stirring.

FLAVOR BOOST: If you are on the STOP plan, sauté 4 ounces sliced shiitake mushrooms along with the leek and tofu.

SUBSTITUTION: For REINTRODUCE, replace the leek with ¼ cup chopped onion.

Serving size: 2 cups Calories: 117; Protein: 8g; Total fat: 6g; Saturated fat: 1g; Carbohydrates: 12g; Fiber: 2g; Sodium: 1342mg

Italian Vegetable Soup

PREP TIME: 10 MINUTES; COOK TIME: 15 MINUTES

Alkalizing vegetables calm your system and fill you up, while kidney beans add protein and heartiness to this delicious savory soup. SERVES 4

30-MINUTE
ONE-POT

1 tablespoon olive oil

1 leek, green part only, chopped and washed (see headnote, page 110)

1 carrot, peeled and chopped

1 zucchini, chopped

1 cup green beans, trimmed and chopped

1 cup canned kidney beans

1 tablespoon dried Italian seasoning

½ teaspoon sea salt

7 cups Simple Vegetable Broth (page 108)

2 tablespoons chopped fresh basil

1. In a large nonstick pot, heat the olive oil over medium-high heat until it shimmers.

2. Add the leek, carrot, and zucchini and cook, stirring occasionally, until the leek is soft, about 5 minutes.

3. Add the green beans, kidney beans, Italian seasoning, salt, and vegetable broth. Bring to a simmer, then lower the heat to medium. Simmer, stirring occasionally, until the green beans are tender, 5 to 7 minutes.

4. Stir in the basil just before serving.

FLAVOR BOOST: Sprinkle each bowl of soup with 1 tablespoon grated Parmesan cheese.

SUBSTITUTION: For REINTRODUCE, replace the leek with ½ onion, chopped.

Serving size: 2 cups Calories: 120; Protein: 5g; Total fat: 4g; Saturated fat: <1g; Carbohydrates: 18g; Fiber: 6g; Sodium: 445mg

Creamy Pumpkin Soup

PREP TIME: 10 MINUTES; COOK TIME: 15 MINUTES

Pumpkin has a sweet earthy flavor that pairs well with sage. Canned pumpkin makes this soup quick and easy, and the soup will store well in the refrigerator for up to 5 days or in the freezer for up to 3 months. Enjoy it with a piece of gluten-free toast for a hearty meal.
SERVES 4

30-MINUTE

1 tablespoon olive oil

1 leek, green part only, finely chopped and washed (see headnote, page 110)

1 cup canned pure pumpkin (not pumpkin pie filling)

3 cups Simple Vegetable Broth (page 108)

1 teaspoon dried sage

½ teaspoon sea salt

½ cup light coconut milk

1 teaspoon cornstarch

1. In a large saucepan, heat the olive oil over medium-high heat until it shimmers.

2. Add the leek and cook, stirring, until soft, about 5 minutes.

3. Add the pumpkin, vegetable broth, sage, and salt. Bring to a simmer and cook for 5 minutes.

4. In a small bowl, whisk together the coconut milk and cornstarch.

5. Remove the pan from the heat and carefully pour the soup into a blender or food processor, along with the coconut milk and cornstarch. Allow the steam to escape through the hole in the blender lid or the food processor feed tube as you blend, to avoid a buildup of pressure. Blend until smooth.

6. Return the soup to the pot and warm over medium heat for 2 minutes, or until thick.

FLAVOR BOOST: Add texture by garnishing each bowl with ½ cup air-popped popcorn or 1 tablespoon pepitas (hulled pumpkin seeds).

SUBSTITUTION: For REINTRODUCE, replace the leek with ¼ onion, chopped.

Serving size: 1 cup Calories: 92; Protein: 2g; Total fat: 5g; Saturated fat: 2g; Carbohydrates: 10g; Fiber: 2g; Sodium: 245mg

Cream of Broccoli Soup

PREP TIME: 10 MINUTES; COOK TIME: 15 MINUTES

In this soup, the broccoli is the star, with all the other ingredients playing supporting roles. Serve alone, or with a slice of gluten-free toast or a few gluten-free crackers on the side.

SERVES 4

30-MINUTE

1 tablespoon olive oil

1 leek, green part only, finely chopped and washed (see headnote, page 110)

3 cups broccoli florets

6 cups Simple Vegetable Broth (page 108)

½ teaspoon sea salt

1 cup lactose-free nonfat milk

1 tablespoon cornstarch

¼ cup lactose-free nonfat plain yogurt, for garnish (optional)

½ cup baby kale, for garnish (optional)

¼ cup microgreens, for garnish (optional)

1. In a large pot, heat the olive oil over medium-high heat until it shimmers.

2. Add the leek and broccoli and cook, stirring, until the leek is soft, about 5 minutes.

3. Add the vegetable broth and salt. Bring to a simmer. Lower the heat to medium and simmer, stirring occasionally, until the broccoli is soft, about 5 minutes.

4. In a small bowl, whisk together the milk and cornstarch. Stir into the soup. Cook for a few minutes more, stirring, until the soup thickens slightly.

5. Thin the yogurt (if using) with a little water. Drizzle it on the soup as a garnish.

6. Garnish with the kale and microgreens (if using)

FLAVOR BOOST: Garnish each bowl of soup with 2 tablespoons grated Cheddar cheese.

SUBSTITUTION: For REINTRODUCE, replace the leek with ½ onion, finely chopped.

Serving size: 2 cups Calories: 127; Protein: 6g; Total fat: 4g; Saturated fat: <1g; Carbohydrates: 19g; Fiber: 4g; Sodium: 401mg

STOP

HEAL

REINTRODUCE

Sweet Potato and Corn Stew

PREP TIME: 10 MINUTES; COOK TIME: 15 MINUTES

This stew is nicely scented with cumin, which pairs well with the sweet, earthy flavor of the sweet potato. Corn adds a nice textural element, while chopped fresh cilantro added at the end imparts fresh, herbal flavors. SERVES 2

30-MINUTE

1 tablespoon olive oil

1 leek, green part only, finely chopped and washed (see headnote, page 110)

2 cups spinach

1 medium sweet potato, peeled and cut into ½-inch cubes (1 cup or less)

½ cup canned or frozen corn

3 cups Simple Vegetable Broth (page 108)

2 teaspoons cornstarch

1 teaspoon dried cumin

½ teaspoon sea salt

1 cup lactose-free nonfat plain yogurt

¼ cup chopped fresh cilantro

½ teaspoon grated lime zest

1. In a large saucepan, heat the olive oil over medium-high heat until it shimmers.

2. Add the leek and cook, stirring occasionally, until soft, about 5 minutes.

3. Add the spinach, sweet potato, and corn.

4. In a bowl, whisk together the vegetable broth, cornstarch, cumin, and salt. Add to the pan and bring to a simmer.

5. Lower the heat to medium. Cook, stirring occasionally, until the sweet potato is soft, about 10 minutes.

6. Stir in the yogurt, cilantro, and lime zest just before serving.

FLAVOR BOOST: Garnish each bowl with ⅛ avocado, chopped.

SUBSTITUTION: For REINTRODUCE, replace the leek with ½ onion, finely chopped.

Serving size: 2 cups Calories: 248; Protein: 8g; Total fat: 8g; Saturated fat: 2g; Carbohydrates: 39g; Fiber: 5g; Sodium: 613mg

Broccoli and Cheese Baked Potato

PREP TIME: 10 MINUTES; COOK TIME: 1 HOUR 30 MINUTES

Baked potatoes take a while to cook, but it's all passive time. You can even cook them ahead and reheat them in the microwave for a minute or two when you're ready to serve them, making this an easy make-ahead meal. SERVES 2

5-INGREDIENT
ONE-PAN

2 small russet potatoes

1 cup broccoli florets

½ teaspoon sea salt

½ cup grated
  Cheddar cheese

1. Preheat the oven to 350°F. Pierce the potatoes several times with a fork.

2. Bake the potatoes on a rimmed baking sheet for 1 hour. Add the broccoli to the pan in a single layer. Continue to roast for 30 minutes, or until the potatoes are soft and the broccoli is tender.

3. Split the potatoes. Season with the salt and top with the broccoli and Cheddar. (Melt the cheese in the microwave for about 45 seconds, if desired.)

FLAVOR BOOST: For HEAL or REINTRODUCE, add a dollop (about 2 tablespoons) of lactose-free nonfat plain yogurt, if desired.

Serving size: 1 potato, ½ cup broccoli Calories: 247; Protein: 11g; Total fat: 10g; Saturated fat: 6g; Carbohydrates: 30g; Fiber: 5g; Sodium: 669mg

STOP

HEAL

REINTRODUCE

Lentil Tacos

PREP TIME: 10 MINUTES; COOK TIME: 15 MINUTES

Lentils make a great taco filling, especially when combined with warm spices such as cumin and coriander. You can heat your tortillas in the oven while cooking the lentils and then put everything on the table so people can assemble their own tacos. SERVES 4

30-MINUTE
ONE-PAN

4 small corn tortillas

1 tablespoon olive oil

1 leek, green part only, chopped and washed (see headnote, page 110)

2 cups canned lentils

¼ cup Simple Vegetable Broth (page 108)

1 teaspoon ground cumin

½ teaspoon ground coriander

½ teaspoon sea salt

¼ avocado, chopped

¼ cup chopped fresh cilantro

1. Preheat the oven to 350°F. Wrap the tortillas in aluminum foil and put them in the oven to warm for 15 minutes.

2. Meanwhile, in a large saucepan, heat the olive oil over medium-high heat until it shimmers. Add the leek and cook until soft, about 5 minutes.

3. Add the lentils, vegetable broth, cumin, coriander, and salt. Bring to a simmer and then lower the heat to medium. Simmer, stirring occasionally, for 5 minutes.

4. To serve, spoon the lentils onto the tortillas, and top with the avocado and cilantro.

FLAVOR BOOST: Replace the avocado with Guacamole (page 207).

Serving size: ½ cup lentils, 1 corn tortilla Calories: 256; Protein: 9g; Total fat: 8g; Saturated fat: 1g; Carbohydrates: 37g; Fiber: 6g; Sodium: 366mg

Pasta with Walnut Pesto

PREP TIME: 10 MINUTES; COOK TIME: 10 MINUTES

If it's pasta you're craving, there are many gluten-free varieties available. Choose your favorite variety and shape here—spaghetti and penne are both great with pesto sauce because the noodles hold the sauce well. SERVES 2

5-INGREDIENT
30-MINUTE

¼ cup tightly packed fresh basil leaves

¼ cup walnuts

¼ cup grated Parmesan cheese

1 tablespoon olive oil

1 teaspoon grated lemon zest

½ teaspoon sea salt

1 cup dry gluten-free penne, cooked according to package instructions and drained

1. In a blender or food processor, combine the basil, walnuts, Parmesan, olive oil, lemon zest, and salt.

2. Pulse 15 to 20 times, until well chopped.

3. Toss the pesto with the hot cooked pasta.

SUBSTITUTION: If you're seeking a more classic pesto, you can replace the walnuts with ¼ cup pine nuts. For REINTRODUCE, add ½ garlic clove, minced, to the pesto.

Serving size: 1 cup pasta, ¼ cup pesto Calories: 293; Protein: 9g; Total fat: 13g; Saturated fat: 3g; Carbohydrates: 38g; Fiber: 2g; Sodium: 598mg

STOP

HEAL

REINTRODUCE

Zucchini and Carrot Frittata

PREP TIME: 10 MINUTES; COOK TIME: 15 MINUTES

Frittatas are delicious for any meal. They also keep well, so it's easy to make them ahead, refrigerate for up to 3 days, and take a portion with you for lunches on the go. SERVES 4

5-INGREDIENT

30-MINUTE

1 tablespoon olive oil

1 carrot, peeled
    and chopped

1 zucchini, grated

4 large eggs

1 tablespoon chopped
    fresh thyme

¼ teaspoon sea salt

1. Preheat the broiler on high.

2. In a large, oven-safe nonstick skillet, heat the olive oil over medium-high heat until it shimmers.

3. Add the carrot and cook, stirring occasionally, until it begins to soften, about 3 minutes.

4. Add the zucchini and cook for 2 minutes.

5. In a medium bowl, whisk the eggs with the thyme and salt.

6. Spread out the vegetables evenly in the bottom of the skillet.

7. Carefully pour the eggs over the top. Lower the heat to medium.

8. Cook until the eggs begin to set around the edges, about 2 minutes. Using a spatula, carefully pull the set eggs away from the sides of the skillet. Tilt the skillet to distribute the uncooked egg into the space you've made. Cook until the eggs set around the edges again, 2 to 3 minutes more.

9. Transfer the skillet to the broiler. Broil until set on top, 2 to 3 minutes.

10. Cut into wedges to serve.

SUBSTITUTION TIP: For REINTRODUCE, sauté ¼ cup chopped onion along with the carrot.

Serving size: ¼ frittata Calories: 116; Protein: 7g; Total fat: 9g; Saturated fat: 2g; Carbohydrates: 4g; Fiber: 1g; Sodium: 195mg

Zucchini Ribbons with Parmesan Cream Sauce

PREP TIME: 10 MINUTES; COOK TIME: 10 MINUTES

It's easy to turn zucchini into noodles, and you don't need any special equipment other than a vegetable peeler. Simply draw your peeler down the length of the zucchini to make ribbons that you can then cook as pasta. SERVES 2

5-INGREDIENT

30-MINUTE

1 tablespoon olive oil

3 small zucchini, cut into ribbons with a vegetable peeler (see headnote)

½ teaspoon sea salt

½ cup lactose-free nonfat milk

¼ cup grated Parmesan cheese

1. In a large, nonstick skillet, heat the olive oil over medium-high heat until it shimmers.

2. Add the zucchini and salt and cook, stirring occasionally, until tender, about 4 minutes.

3. While the zucchini cooks, heat the milk in a small saucepan over medium heat. When it simmers, whisk in the Parmesan.

4. Cook the milk mixture, stirring, until smooth. Toss with the cooked zucchini.

FLAVOR BOOST: Add ¼ cup chopped fresh basil when you mix the zucchini and pasta.

Serving size: 1 cup zucchini, ¼ cup sauce Calories: 177; Protein: 11g; Total fat: 11g; Saturated fat: 3g; Carbohydrates: 12g; Fiber: 2g; Sodium: 681mg

STOP

HEAL

REINTRODUCE

Asian Veggie and Tofu Stir-Fry

PREP TIME: 10 MINUTES; COOK TIME: 10 MINUTES

The great thing about stir-fries is you can change veggies depending on your flavor preferences. They're also super quick, and they are delicious by themselves or served on a bed of hot rice or soba (buckwheat) noodles. SERVES 2

**30-MINUTE
ONE-PAN**

¼ cup Simple Vegetable
  Broth (page 108)

1 teaspoon miso paste

½ teaspoon grated
  fresh ginger

½ teaspoon grated
  orange zest

½ teaspoon sea salt

1 tablespoon olive oil

6 ounces extra-firm tofu,
  cut into ½-inch cubes

1 leek, green part only,
  chopped and washed
  (see headnote, page 110)

2 carrots, peeled
  and chopped

2 cups chopped bok choy

1. In a small bowl, whisk together the broth, miso, ginger, orange zest, and salt. Set aside.

2. In a large, nonstick skillet, heat the olive oil over medium-high heat until it shimmers.

3. Add the tofu, leek, carrots, and bok choy. Cook, stirring occasionally, until the veggies begin to brown, 5 to 7 minutes.

4. Add the reserved sauce and bring to a simmer. Cook, stirring, until the sauce thickens, 3 to 4 minutes more.

FLAVOR BOOST: Add ¼ cup chopped fresh cilantro just before serving and garnish with 2 tablespoons chopped roasted peanuts.

Serving size: 2 cups Calories: 206; Protein: 11g; Total fat: 12g; Saturated fat: 2g; Carbohydrates: 17g; Fiber: 4g; Sodium: 681mg

Soba Noodles with Peanut Butter Sauce

PREP TIME: 10 MINUTES; COOK TIME: 10 MINUTES

If you like Thai-inspired peanut sauce, this dish will satisfy your craving. The peanut butter sauce has ginger, miso, and cilantro, which add a savory Asian flavor to soba (buckwheat) noodles. SERVES 2

30-MINUTE
ONE-PAN

¼ cup peanut butter

¼ cup light coconut milk

1 teaspoon miso paste

1 teaspoon grated
   fresh ginger

2 tablespoons chopped
   fresh cilantro

Water or Simple
   Vegetable Broth
   (page 108) (optional)

2 ounces soba
   (buckwheat) noodles,
   cooked according to
   package instructions
   and drained

1. In a small saucepan, combine the peanut butter, coconut milk, miso, ginger, and cilantro. Cook over medium-high heat, stirring, until melted and blended. Thin with a little water or broth if needed.

2. Toss with the hot noodles.

SUBSTITUTION: If you can't find soba noodles, you can use an equal amount of gluten-free spaghetti or angel hair pasta. For REINTRODUCE, add ½ garlic clove, minced, to the peanut butter mixture.

Serving size: 1 cup noodles, ¼ cup peanut butter sauce
Calories: 311; Protein: 13g; Total fat: 19g; Saturated fat: 5g;
Carbohydrates: 27g; Fiber: 3g; Sodium: 263mg

Brown Rice and Peanut Lettuce Wraps

PREP TIME: 10 MINUTES; COOK TIME: 10 MINUTES

Using precooked brown rice allows this dish to come together quickly. You can find precooked brown rice in the rice or freezer section at the grocery store, or cook some yourself and store 1-cup portions in resealable bags in the freezer for up to 3 months.
SERVES 2

30-MINUTE
ONE-PAN

1 tablespoon olive oil

1 leek, green part only, finely chopped and washed (see headnote, page 110)

3 ounces extra-firm tofu, cut into ¼-inch cubes

1½ cups cooked brown rice

2 tablespoons crunchy peanut butter

1 tablespoon grated fresh ginger

¼ cup Simple Vegetable Broth (page 108)

½ teaspoon sea salt

2 tablespoons chopped fresh cilantro

4 large lettuce leaves

1. In a nonstick skillet, heat the olive oil over medium-high heat until it shimmers. Add the leek and tofu and cook, stirring, until the leek is soft, about 5 minutes.

2. Add the rice, peanut butter, ginger, broth, and salt. Cook, stirring constantly, until well blended and hot, about 4 minutes.

3. Stir in the cilantro.

4. Spoon the rice mixture into the lettuce leaves, roll them up, and serve.

FLAVOR BOOST: For extra texture, add 1 tablespoon chopped roasted peanuts to each lettuce wrap.

SUBSTITUTE: For REINTRODUCE, replace the leek with 3 chopped scallions.

Serving size: 1 cup rice, 2 lettuce leaves Calories: 445; Protein: 14g; Total fat: 27g; Saturated fat: 4g; Carbohydrates: 38g; Fiber: 4g; Sodium: 603mg

Vegetable and Tofu Fried Rice

PREP TIME: 10 MINUTES; COOK TIME: 10 MINUTES

This satisfying fried rice dish keeps well in the refrigerator for up to 3 days or in the freezer for up to 3 months, and it reheats well in the microwave. Use precooked brown rice (you'll find it in the rice section at the grocery store) to make this a super quick and easy meal. SERVES 4

30-MINUTE

1 tablespoon olive oil

1 leek, green part only, finely chopped and washed (see headnote, page 110)

1 carrot, peeled and chopped

½ cup broccoli florets

3 ounces extra-firm tofu, cut into ¼-inch pieces

1 tablespoon grated fresh ginger

3 cups cooked brown rice

¼ cup Simple Vegetable Broth (page 108)

1 teaspoon miso paste

1. In a nonstick skillet, heat the olive oil over medium-high heat until it shimmers. Add the leek, carrot, broccoli, tofu, and ginger and cook, stirring, until the veggies are soft, about 5 minutes.

2. Add the rice.

3. In a small bowl, whisk together the broth and miso. Add to the rice.

4. Cook, stirring, until warmed through, 3 to 4 minutes more.

FLAVOR BOOST: If you're on STOP, add ¼ cup cooked peas to the rice. You can also add ¼ cup edamame to the rice when you add the other vegetables.

Serving size: 1 cup Calories: 189; Protein: 5g; Total fat: 6g; Saturated fat: 1g; Carbohydrates: 30g; Fiber: 2g; Sodium: 77mg

STOP

HEAL

REINTRODUCE

Butternut Risotto

PREP TIME: 5 MINUTES; COOK TIME: 20 MINUTES

Risotto takes a lot of stirring, but it's actually pretty easy to make. This recipe features sweet, earthy butternut squash with creamy rice and just a hint of Parmesan for a really tasty meal. Store for up to 3 days in the refrigerator and reheat in the microwave.
SERVES 2

30-MINUTE

2 cups Simple Vegetable Broth (page 108)

1 tablespoon olive oil

1 cup cubed butternut squash

½ cup Arborio rice

1 teaspoon dried thyme

½ teaspoon sea salt

¼ cup grated Parmesan cheese

1. In a medium saucepan, heat the broth over medium-low heat and keep warm.

2. In a large saucepan, heat the olive oil over medium-high heat until it shimmers. Add the squash and cook, stirring, until it starts to brown, about 4 minutes.

3. Add the rice and thyme. Cook, stirring, for 1 minute.

4. One ladleful at a time, add the hot broth, stirring constantly. As the rice starts to look dry, ladle in more broth until the rice is tender. This process will take about 15 minutes total.

5. Turn off the heat and stir in the salt and Parmesan.

SUBSTITUTION: To make this work for HEAL or REINTRODUCE, reduce the butternut squash to ½ cup. For REINTRODUCE, add ½ onion, finely chopped, and cook it with the squash.

Serving size: 1½ cups Calories: 196; Protein: 7g; Total fat: 10g; Saturated fat: 3g; Carbohydrates: 22g; Fiber: 3g; Sodium: 622mg

Brown Rice and Tofu with Kale

PREP TIME: 10 MINUTES; COOK TIME: 15 MINUTES

Using precooked rice in this recipe allows you to get it on the table quickly. If you prefer a firmer tofu, remove the tofu from its carton, put it in a colander in the sink, and place a plate with weights (such as canned food) over the top. Allow it to sit for 30 minutes while the weights and plate press out some of the water, which will give it a denser texture and a firmer bite. SERVES 2

STOP

HEAL

REINTRODUCE

30-MINUTE
ONE-PAN

1 tablespoon olive oil

½ leek, green part only, chopped and washed (see headnote, page 110)

1 cup stemmed and chopped kale

1 carrot, peeled and chopped

1 fennel bulb, cored and chopped

1 teaspoon dried oregano

1 cup Simple Vegetable Broth (page 108)

1½ cups cooked brown rice

½ teaspoon sea salt

½ teaspoon grated orange zest

1. In a large saucepan, heat the olive oil over medium-high heat until it shimmers. Add the leek, kale, carrot, fennel, and oregano. Cook, stirring occasionally, until the vegetables are soft, about 5 minutes.

2. Add the broth, rice, and salt. Cook, stirring, for 2 minutes, or until the broth reduces.

3. Stir in the orange zest.

SUBSTITUTION: If you can't find fennel, substitute 1 medium zucchini, chopped. For REINTRODUCE, substitute ½ onion, chopped, for the leek.

Calories: 254; Protein: 5g; Total fat: 8g; Saturated fat: 1g; Carbohydrates: 43g; Fiber: 6g; Sodium: 582mg

Seasoned Tofu with Chimichurri

PREP TIME: 10 MINUTES; COOK TIME: 10 MINUTES

Use extra-firm tofu for this recipe. For an even firmer texture, drain the tofu for 30 minutes in a colander with a plate with weights set on top of it before cutting into slices and grilling. Serve with a side of steamed rice, or serve the tofu with a salad or steamed veggie.

SERVES 2

5-INGREDIENT
30-MINUTE

½ teaspoon dried oregano

½ teaspoon ground cumin

½ teaspoon ground coriander

½ teaspoon sea salt

6 ounces extra-firm tofu, cut into four slices

1 tablespoon olive oil

¼ cup Oregano and Parsley Chimichurri (page 205)

1. In a small bowl, combine the oregano, cumin, coriander, and salt.

2. Sprinkle the spice rub on both sides of the tofu slices.

3. In a large nonstick skillet, heat the olive oil over medium-high heat until it shimmers.

4. Add the tofu and cook until browned, about 5 minutes per side.

5. Serve topped with the chimichurri.

FLAVOR BOOST: Add 1 teaspoon grated lemon zest to the spice rub.

Serving size: 3 ounces tofu, 2 tablespoons chimichurri
Calories: 183; Protein: 7g; Total fat: 18g; Saturated fat: 3g; Carbohydrates: 2g; Fiber: 1g; Sodium: 479mg

Grilled Eggplant Burgers

PREP TIME: 10 MINUTES; COOK TIME: 15 MINUTES

Eggplant can be bitter, so if you prefer it a bit less so, take the extra step of draining the liquid from the slices. To do this, put the eggplant slices in a colander in the sink and sprinkle them liberally with sea salt. Allow them to sit for about 20 minutes to allow the bitter liquid to drain. Then rinse away the salt and pat the slices dry. Proceed with the recipe as written. SERVES 2

5-INGREDIENT

30-MINUTE

1 tablespoon olive oil

1 teaspoon ground cumin

1 teaspoon dried oregano

½ teaspoon sea salt

2 (¼- to ½-inch-thick) eggplant slices

2 gluten-free hamburger buns

¼ cup Lemon Yogurt Sauce (page 199)

1. Heat an indoor or outdoor grill to high.

2. In a small bowl, stir together the olive oil, cumin, oregano, and salt.

3. Brush the oil mixture on both sides of the eggplant slices. Brush any remaining mixture on the inside of the gluten-free buns.

4. Grill the eggplant slices for 5 to 6 minutes per side, until browned.

5. Grill the buns until toasted, about 1 minute.

6. Assemble the burgers and serve topped with the yogurt sauce.

FLAVOR BOOST: Add crisp lettuce to the bun and, if you are in REINTRODUCE and can tolerate tomatoes, a slice of tomato.

Serving size: 1 burger, 2 tablespoons sauce Calories: 237; Protein: 3g; Total fat: 13g; Saturated fat: 2g; Carbohydrates: 32g; Fiber: 7g; Sodium: 699mg

HEAL

REINTRODUCE

Pesto Grilled Cheese

PREP TIME: 5 MINUTES; COOK TIME: 5 MINUTES

*Grilled cheese is the ultimate comfort food. Serve it with Creamy Pumpkin Soup
(page 112) for a classic comfort meal that will remind you of childhood. While this recipe
calls for Cheddar cheese, you can also use Swiss. Grating the cheese makes it melt evenly
for the perfect sandwich.* SERVES 2

5-INGREDIENT
30-MINUTE
ONE-PAN

2 slices gluten-free
   sandwich bread

1 tablespoon unsalted
   grass-fed butter, at room
   temperature

2 tablespoons Walnut-
   Basil Pesto (page 201)

¼ cup grated
   Cheddar cheese

1. Preheat a medium nonstick skillet over
medium-high heat.

2. Brush one side of each bread slice with the butter.
Spread the other side of each piece with the pesto.

3. Place one slice of bread, butter-side down, in the skillet. Top with the Cheddar and the second slice of bread,
butter-side up.

4. Cook until the bread browns, about 3 minutes. Flip
and cook for an additional 3 minutes to brown the other
side. Cut the sandwich in half to serve.

FLAVOR BOOST: Add a pinch of flavored salt, such as
smoked salt or truffle salt, to the melted butter before you
brush it on the bread.

Serving size: ½ sandwich Calories: 274; Protein: 6g; Total
fat: 20g; Saturated fat: 8g; Carbohydrates: 24g; Fiber: 1g;
Sodium: 414mg

Fried Egg Sandwich

PREP TIME: 5 MINUTES; COOK TIME: 10 MINUTES

If you're looking for a quick and flavorful sandwich and you're an egg lover, then it doesn't get much better than a fried egg sandwich. The sandwich is simplicity at its finest, but the egg yolk soaks the toast to make a really satisfying sandwich. SERVES 1

5-INGREDIENT
30-MINUTE
ONE-PAN

3 teaspoons unsalted grass-fed butter, at room temperature, divided

1 large egg

Pinch sea salt

2 slices gluten-free bread, toasted

1. In a small nonstick skillet, heat 1 teaspoon of butter over medium heat until it melts, swirling the skillet to coat with the butter.

2. Carefully crack the egg into the butter. Season with the salt.

3. Cook until the egg just sets, about 4 minutes. Carefully flip the egg. Turn off the heat and allow the egg to sit in the warm skillet for 45 seconds more.

4. Spread the toast with the remaining 2 teaspoons of butter. Carefully transfer the egg to one slice of bread and top it with the other.

SUBSTITUTION: You can replace the butter with an equal amount of olive oil.

Serving size: 1 sandwich Calories: 411; Protein: 10g; Total fat: 25g; Saturated fat: 15g; Carbohydrates: 40g; Fiber: 2g; Sodium: 924mg

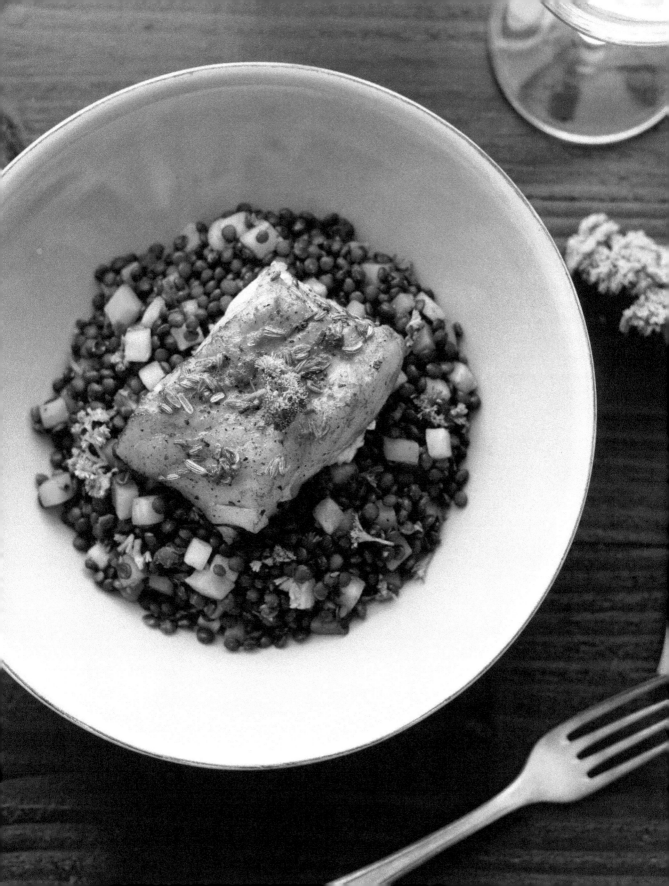

7

Seafood and Poultry

Crab Cakes with Tartar Sauce 132

Miso-Glazed Scallops 133

Breaded Crispy Shrimp 134

Steamer Clams with Fennel 135

Halibut and Veggie Packets 136

Tilapia with Cantaloupe Salsa 137

Easy Tuna Melt 138

Maple-Glazed Salmon 139

Salmon and Lentils 140

Fish Tacos with Guacamole 141

Fisherman's Stew 142

Chicken Noodle Soup 143

Baked Chicken Tenders 144

Oven-Fried Chicken 145

Quick Chicken and Veggie Stir-Fry 146

One-Pot Chicken Stew 147

Easy Turkey Burgers 148

Turkey Meatballs 149

Turkey Meatloaf Muffins 150

Turkey and Spinach Rollatini 151

Salmon and Lentils, page 140

Crab Cakes with Tartar Sauce

PREP TIME: 15 MINUTES; COOK TIME: 10 MINUTES

The trick to binding these bread crumb–free crab cakes is a shrimp mousse, which also adds tremendous flavor to the crab cakes. Serve them with a simple salad for a complete meal. SERVES 2

30-MINUTE

1 cup cooked baby shrimp

¼ cup lactose-free nonfat plain yogurt

1 tablespoon chopped fresh dill

1 teaspoon grated lemon zest

½ teaspoon sea salt

2 cups lump crabmeat, picked over

1 tablespoon olive oil

¼ cup Tartar Sauce (page 197)

1. In a blender or food processor, combine the shrimp, yogurt, dill, lemon zest, and salt. Blend until smooth.

2. Spoon into a medium bowl. Carefully fold in the crabmeat until well combined. Form into four patties.

3. In a large nonstick skillet, heat the oil over medium-high heat until it shimmers.

4. Add the patties. Cook until browned, 4 to 5 minutes per side.

5. Serve topped with the tartar sauce.

FLAVOR BOOST: For added crunch, add ¼ cup finely diced fennel to the crab cakes when you mix in the crab.

SUBSTITUTE: For REINTRODUCE, you can add 2 finely chopped scallions when you add the crab.

Serving size: 2 cakes, 2 tablespoons tartar sauce Calories: 231; Protein: 31g; Total fat: 9g; Saturated fat: 1g; Carbohydrates: 5g; Fiber: <1g; Sodium: 1149mg

Miso-Glazed Scallops

PREP TIME: 5 MINUTES; COOK TIME: 10 MINUTES

When selecting sea scallops, opt for those that have a slightly sweet and briny, but not fishy, odor. To prepare the scallops, you'll need to remove the tendon that runs along and bulges from the side of the scallop. To do this, use a sharp paring knife to cut it away.

SERVES 2

5-INGREDIENT

30-MINUTE

¼ cup pure maple syrup

1 teaspoon miso paste

½ teaspoon sea salt

8 sea scallops,
   tendons removed

1 tablespoon unsalted
   grass-fed butter

1. In a small bowl, whisk together the maple syrup, miso, and salt.

2. Brush the scallops with the mixture.

3. In a large nonstick skillet, melt the butter over medium-high heat.

4. Add the scallops and cook until just opaque, about 3 minutes per side.

FLAVOR BOOST: Add 1 teaspoon grated orange zest to the miso mixture.

Serving size: 4 scallops Calories: 214; Protein: 11g; Total fat: 7g; Saturated fat: 4g; Carbohydrates: 30g; Fiber: <1g; Sodium: 680mg

Breaded Crispy Shrimp

PREP TIME: 5 MINUTES; COOK TIME: 12 MINUTES

It's easy to make your own gluten-free bread crumbs. Simple remove the crust from three or four slices of gluten-free bread and allow the slices to sit out overnight on the counter to get slightly stale. Then pulse them in a food processor or blender 10 to 20 times to make bread crumbs. You may also be able to find them commercially. SERVES 2

5-INGREDIENT
30-MINUTE

1 cup gluten-free
   bread crumbs

1 teaspoon sea salt

1 teaspoon dried thyme

½ teaspoon
   ground mustard

2 large eggs

2 cups medium raw
   shrimp, peeled and
   deveined, tails removed

1. Preheat the oven to 400°F.

2. In a small bowl, combine the bread crumbs, salt, thyme, and mustard, mixing well.

3. Beat the eggs in a separate bowl.

4. Dip each shrimp first into the beaten eggs and then into the bread crumbs, tapping off any excess coating. Place the shrimp in a single layer on a rimmed baking sheet.

5. Bake, turning once, until the shrimp are golden brown, 10 to 12 minutes.

FLAVOR BOOST: Serve with Tartar Sauce (page 197).

Serving size: 1 cup shrimp Calories: 307; Protein: 42g; Total fat: 8g; Saturated fat: 2g; Carbohydrates: 12g; Fiber: 1g; Sodium: 1358mg

Steamer Clams with Fennel

PREP TIME: 10 MINUTES; COOK TIME: 10 MINUTES

One pound of steamer clams per person may seem like a lot, but that's mostly shell, so portions remain in control. Serve with a crusty gluten-free bread (for dipping in the delicious broth) and a side of steamed vegetables for a satisfying summer meal. SERVES 2

30-MINUTE
ONE-POT

1 tablespoon unsalted grass-fed butter

1 fennel bulb, cored and chopped, fronds reserved

1 leek, green part only, chopped and washed (see headnote, page 110)

2 pounds steamer clams

2 cups Simple Vegetable Broth (page 108)

Grated zest of 1 lemon

½ teaspoon sea salt

1. In a large pot, melt the butter over medium-high heat.

2. Add the fennel bulb and leek and cook, stirring occasionally, until soft, about 5 minutes.

3. Add the steamer clams, broth, lemon zest, and salt. Cover and cook until the clams open, about 5 minutes. (Discard any that did not open.)

4. Chop the fennel fronds and stir them into the broth.

FLAVOR BOOST: If you're in the REINTRODUCE phase and you tolerate tomatoes, stir in about ½ cup chopped fresh tomatoes when you add the broth.

SUBSTITUTE: Replace the leek with ½ onion, finely chopped.

Serving size: 1 pound clams Calories: 164; Protein: 11g; Total fat: 7g; Saturated fat: 4g; Carbohydrates: 17g; Fiber: 4g; Sodium: 576mg

Halibut and Veggie Packets

PREP TIME: 10 MINUTES; COOK TIME: 20 MINUTES

Cooking halibut with vegetables in parchment paper packets keeps the fish tender and flavorful and steams the vegetables to the perfect level of tenderness. You can cook these packets in your oven or put them on the grill in the summer. SERVES 2

30-MINUTE
ONE-PAN

1 zucchini, sliced

6 ounces halibut, halved

1 teaspoon grated
   lemon zest

1 teaspoon dried dill

½ teaspoon sea salt

2 tablespoons unsalted
   grass-fed butter, cut into
   two pats

1. Preheat the oven to 350°F.

2. Place two 12-inch squares of parchment paper on a rimmed baking sheet.

3. Divide the zucchini slices between the squares and top each with a piece of halibut. Sprinkle each with half of the lemon zest, dill, and salt. Top each with a pat of butter.

4. Fold the squares into packets and seal the edges with narrow folds. Place the baking sheet in the oven and bake until the halibut is flaky, about 20 minutes.

SUBSTITUTION: If you can't find halibut, you can substitute salmon, trout, cod, or another white fish. If you're following REINTRODUCE, add ¼ tomato, chopped, to each of the packets.

Serving size: 1 packet Calories: 228; Protein: 24g; Total fat: 14g; Saturated fat: 8g; Carbohydrates: 4g; Fiber: 1g; Sodium: 539mg

Tilapia with Cantaloupe Salsa

PREP TIME: 10 MINUTES; COOK TIME: 15 MINUTES

Fish with a fresh fruit salsa makes a lovely summer dish. While this recipe recommends baking the fish in the oven, if it's a nice day you can cook the fish on the grill. Be on the lookout for pin bones and use a pair of tweezers to remove any quickly and easily.

SERVES 2

5-INGREDIENT
30-MINUTE
ONE-PAN

2 (3-ounce) tilapia fillets

1 tablespoon olive oil

½ teaspoon dried cumin

½ teaspoon sea salt

**½ cup Cantaloupe Salsa
  (page 206)**

1. Preheat the oven to 425°F.

2. Place the fish fillets on a rimmed baking sheet. Brush with the olive oil and sprinkle with the cumin and salt.

3. Bake until the fish flakes, 10 to 15 minutes.

4. Top each fillet with half of the salsa.

SUBSTITUTION: If you can't find tilapia, try cod or salmon in its place.

Serving size: 3 ounces tilapia, ¼ cup salsa Calories: 152; Protein: 17g; Total fat: 8g; Saturated fat: 1g; Carbohydrates: 4g; Fiber: <1g; Sodium: 997mg

Easy Tuna Melt

PREP TIME: 10 MINUTES; COOK TIME: 5 MINUTES

Who doesn't love a tuna melt? This classic sandwich is GERD-friendly, quick, and satisfying. You can add an herb for extra flavor (see Flavor Boost), or keep it classic by sticking with just the basics of tuna, dressing, cheese, and bread. SERVES 2

5-INGREDIENT

30-MINUTE

6 ounces water-packed tuna, drained

3 tablespoons lactose-free nonfat plain yogurt

½ teaspoon sea salt

2 slices gluten-free sandwich bread, toasted

½ cup grated Cheddar cheese

1. Preheat the broiler on high.

2. In a small bowl, combine the tuna, yogurt, and salt.

3. Place the toasted bread on a rimmed baking sheet and spread each with half of the tuna mixture.

4. Top with the Cheddar.

5. Broil until the cheese melts, 3 to 4 minutes.

FLAVOR BOOST: Add 1 tablespoon chopped fresh dill or tarragon and ½ teaspoon grated lemon or orange zest to the yogurt.

Serving size: 1 sandwich Calories: 345; Protein: 32g; Total fat: 14g; Saturated fat: 7g; Carbohydrates: 22g; Fiber: 1g; Sodium: 1016mg

Maple-Glazed Salmon

PREP TIME: 10 MINUTES; COOK TIME: 15 MINUTES

This orange, maple, and miso glaze pairs well with flavorful salmon. Serve this main dish with a side of steamed broccoli and ¼ cup of cooked brown rice for a satisfying and delicious meal. Or, try serving it with Sweet Potato Hash (page 81). SERVES 2

5-INGREDIENT

30-MINUTE

¼ cup Simple Vegetable Broth (page 108)

¼ cup pure maple syrup

1 teaspoon miso paste

1 teaspoon grated orange zest

½ teaspoon sea salt

2 (3-ounce) salmon fillets

1. Preheat the oven to 400°F.

2. In a medium bowl, whisk together the broth, maple syrup, miso, orange zest, and salt. Marinate the salmon in it for 5 minutes, turning the fish once.

3. Place the salmon on a rimmed baking sheet. Bake until the salmon is flaky, about 15 minutes.

FLAVOR BOOST: Add 1 tablespoon chopped fresh tarragon to the marinade.

Serving size: 3 ounces salmon Calories: 259; Protein: 17g; Total fat: 9g; Saturated fat: 2g; Carbohydrates: 27g; Fiber: <1g; Sodium: 629mg

Salmon and Lentils

PREP TIME: 10 MINUTES; COOK TIME: 15 MINUTES

Using canned lentils means this dish comes together quickly, and it's packed with nutritious omega-3 fatty acids and plenty of fiber. SERVES 2

30-MINUTE

2 (3-ounce) salmon fillets

½ teaspoon ground cumin

½ teaspoon sea
  salt, divided

1 tablespoon olive oil

1 carrot, peeled
  and chopped

1 parsnip, peeled
  and chopped

1 cup canned lentils,
  drained and rinsed

1 tablespoon chopped
  fresh dill

1 tablespoon chopped
  fresh curly-leaf parsley,
  for garnish (optional)

1. Preheat the oven to 400°F.

2. Season the salmon with the cumin and ¼ teaspoon of sea salt.

3. Place the salmon on a rimmed baking sheet. Bake until the salmon is flaky, about 15 minutes.

4. Meanwhile, heat the oil in a small skillet over medium-high heat until it shimmers.

5. Add the carrot and parsnip and cook, stirring occasionally, until brown, about 5 minutes.

6. Add the lentils and the remaining ¼ teaspoon of sea salt. Cook until heated through, about 4 minutes more.

7. Stir in the dill.

8. Serve the salmon spooned over the lentils.

9. Garnish with parsley (if using).

FLAVOR BOOST: Add the zest of ½ orange to the lentils.

Serving size: 3 ounces salmon, ½ cup lentils Calories: 358; Protein: 24g; Total fat: 17g; Saturated fat: 3g; Carbohydrates: 30g; Fiber: 7g; Sodium: 726mg

Fish Tacos with Guacamole

PREP TIME: 10 MINUTES; COOK TIME: 15 MINUTES

Tacos are always a family favorite, so if you share this recipe with your family, give them some salsa and sour cream to round out their portions. It's a great way to prepare only one meal but allow everyone to eat what they choose. SERVES 4

30-MINUTE

4 corn tortillas

1 tablespoon olive oil

8 ounces cod, skinned and cut into ½-inch pieces

1 teaspoon grated lime zest

1 teaspoon ground cumin

½ teaspoon ground coriander

½ teaspoon sea salt

1 cup grated Cheddar cheese

½ cup chopped fresh cilantro

½ cup Guacamole (page 207)

1. Preheat the oven to 350°F. Wrap the tortillas in aluminum foil and put them in the oven to warm for 15 minutes.

2. Meanwhile, in a large nonstick skillet, heat the oil over medium-high heat until it shimmers.

3. Add the cod, lime zest, cumin, coriander, and salt. Cook, stirring, until the cod is opaque and firm, about 5 minutes.

4. To assemble the tacos, divide the cod among the warmed corn tortillas. Top each with some Cheddar, cilantro, and guacamole.

SUBSTITUTION: For HEAL, replace the guacamole with ⅛ avocado, chopped, for each taco.

Serving size: 1 taco Calories: 312; Protein: 23g; Total fat: 19g; Saturated fat: 8g; Carbohydrates: 14g; Fiber: 4g; Sodium: 699mg

Fisherman's Stew

PREP TIME: 10 MINUTES; COOK TIME: 20 MINUTES

This hearty stew is a wonderful and warming meal for a chilly fall or winter evening. Substitute any fish you like for the salmon; if you're looking for something a bit lighter, you can use a white fish such as cod, or if you prefer shellfish, you can substitute shrimp—this stew is highly customizable to your personal tastes. SERVES 2

30-MINUTE

1 tablespoon olive oil

1 leek, green part only, chopped and washed (see headnote, page 110)

1 fennel bulb, cored and chopped, fronds reserved

6 ounces salmon, skinned and cut into ½-inch pieces

½ teaspoon cornstarch

3 cups Simple Vegetable Broth (page 108)

6 baby red potatoes, quartered

2 carrots, peeled and chopped

½ teaspoon sea salt

1. In a large pot, heat the oil over medium-high heat until it shimmers. Add the leek and fennel. Cook, stirring occasionally, until the vegetables start to brown, about 5 minutes.

2. Add the salmon and cook, stirring, for 3 minutes more.

3. In a small bowl, whisk the cornstarch into the broth, then add it to the pot, along with the potatoes, carrots, and salt.

4. Cook, stirring occasionally, until the potatoes are soft, about 10 minutes.

5. Chop the fennel fronds and stir them into the stew.

FLAVOR BOOST: Add 1 teaspoon dried thyme and 1 teaspoon grated orange zest when you add the broth.

SUBSTITUTION: For REINTRODUCE, replace the leek with ½ onion, finely chopped.

Serving size: 2 cups Calories: 420; Protein: 22g; Total fat: 17g; Saturated fat: 23g; Carbohydrates: 49g; Fiber: 9g; Sodium: 639mg

Chicken Noodle Soup

PREP TIME: 10 MINUTES; COOK TIME: 20 MINUTES

Using a rotisserie chicken from the grocery store speeds up the time it takes to make this soup. Then, you can use any leftover chicken for meals during the week and use the carcass for making Poultry Broth (page 195). SERVES 4

30-MINUTE
ONE-PAN

1 tablespoon olive oil

1 leek, green part only, chopped and washed (see headnote, page 110)

1 carrot, peeled and chopped

1 celery stalk, chopped

8 cups Poultry Broth (page 195)

1 teaspoon dried thyme

1 teaspoon sea salt

1 ounce gluten-free spaghetti

8 ounces rotisserie chicken meat, skin removed

1. In a large pot, heat the oil over medium-high heat until it shimmers. Add the leek, carrot, and celery. Cook, stirring occasionally, until the vegetables start to brown, about 5 minutes.

2. Add the broth, thyme, and salt. Bring to a boil and add the spaghetti. Cook, stirring occasionally, until the spaghetti is soft, about 9 minutes.

3. Stir in the chicken and cook for 5 more minutes.

SUBSTITUTION: For REINTRODUCE, replace the leek with ½ onion, chopped, or add ½ teaspoon garlic powder when you add the thyme.

Serving size: 2 cups Calories: 226; Protein: 22g; Total fat: 6g; Saturated fat: 1g; Carbohydrates: 21g; Fiber: 1g; Sodium: 736mg

STOP

HEAL

REINTRODUCE

STOP

HEAL

REINTRODUCE

Baked Chicken Tenders

PREP TIME: 10 MINUTES; COOK TIME: 20 MINUTES

The trick to flavorful baked tenders is a well-seasoned bread crumb mixture. Adding plenty of herbs and a little more salt than normal helps make the bread crumbs flavorful and makes these tenders super tasty. Serve with Creamy Herbed Dressing (page 200) for dipping and Mashed Potatoes (page 101) for a full meal. SERVES 2

30-MINUTE

Nonstick cooking spray

1 cup gluten-free
bread crumbs

1 tablespoon
dried oregano

2 teaspoons dried thyme

¾ teaspoon sea salt

½ teaspoon
ground mustard

2 large eggs

6 ounces boneless,
skinless chicken breast,
cut into eight strips

1. Preheat the oven to 425°F. Coat a rimmed baking sheet with nonstick cooking spray.

2. In a bowl, mix the bread crumbs, oregano, thyme, salt, and mustard.

3. In a separate bowl, beat the eggs.

4. Dip the chicken strips into the eggs and then into the bread crumb mixture, tapping off any excess coating.

5. Place the chicken tenders in a single layer on the prepared baking sheet. Bake until the chicken is golden brown, 15 to 20 minutes.

SUBSTITUTION: You can also make fish sticks or turkey tenders using this recipe. Just replace the chicken with an equal amount of cod or boneless, skinless turkey breast.

Serving size: 4 tenders Calories: 233; Protein: 26g; Total fat: 7g; Saturated fat: 2g; Carbohydrates: 16g; Fiber: 2g; Sodium: 924mg

Oven-Fried Chicken

PREP TIME: 10 MINUTES; COOK TIME: 1 HOUR

Craving fried chicken? Try this oven-baked recipe for chicken legs. Serve with a steamed veggie, steamed rice, or oven-baked Sweet Potato French Fries (page 96). To make this more flavorful, add garlic and spice (see Flavor Boost). SERVES 4

5-INGREDIENT

1 cup gluten-free
  bread crumbs

1 tablespoon dried thyme

¾ teaspoon sea salt

3 large eggs

4 whole chicken legs

1. Preheat the oven to 350°F. Line a rimmed baking sheet with parchment paper or grease the baking sheet.

2. In a bowl, mix the bread crumbs, thyme, and salt.

3. In a separate bowl, beat the eggs.

4. Dip the chicken legs into the eggs and then into the bread crumb mixture, tapping off any excess coating.

5. Place in a single layer on the prepared baking sheet. Bake, turning once, until the chicken is golden brown, about 1 hour.

FLAVOR BOOST: If you're in REINTRODUCE, add 1 teaspoon garlic powder and 1 teaspoon ground mustard to the bread crumbs for extra seasoning.

Serving size: 1 chicken leg Calories: 293; Protein: 26g; Total fat: 18g; Saturated fat: 5g; Carbohydrates: 7g; Fiber: 0g; Sodium: 541mg

STOP

HEAL

REINTRODUCE

Quick Chicken and Veggie Stir-Fry

PREP TIME: 10 MINUTES; COOK TIME: 10 MINUTES

Serve this stir-fry by itself or with ¼ cup of brown rice or soba (buckwheat) noodles for a quick and easy dinner. If you're feeling creative, try using different vegetables to change the flavor profile and texture. SERVES 2

30-MINUTE
ONE-PAN

1 tablespoon olive oil

6 ounces boneless,
  skinless chicken breast,
  cut into ½-inch pieces

1 leek, green part only,
  chopped and washed
  (see headnote, page 110)

2 carrots, peeled
  and chopped

2 cups chopped bok choy

½ cup edamame, thawed
  if frozen

¼ cup Stir-Fry Sauce
  (page 204)

1 tablespoon chopped
  fresh cilantro

1. In a large nonstick skillet or wok, heat the oil over medium-high heat until it shimmers.

2. Add the chicken, leek, carrots, bok choy, and edamame. Cook, stirring occasionally, until the chicken is cooked and the veggies tender, about 5 minutes.

3. Add the stir-fry sauce. Cook, stirring occasionally, for 4 minutes more.

4. Stir in the cilantro.

SUBSTITUTION: If you can't find edamame (look in the freezer aisle), you can substitute an equal amount of green beans. For REINTRODUCE, replace the leek with 3 chopped scallions.

Serving size: 2 cups Calories: 323; Protein: 28g; Total fat: 14g; Saturated fat: 2g; Carbohydrates: 24g; Fiber: 6g; Sodium: 312mg

One-Pot Chicken Stew

PREP TIME: 10 MINUTES; COOK TIME: 20 MINUTES

This stew keeps well in the refrigerator or freezer, and you can reheat it in the microwave or on the stove top. So this is a great recipe to make ahead on a weekend when you know you've got a busy week coming up and you'll need quick meals at the ready. SERVES 4

30-MINUTE

1 tablespoon olive oil

6 ounces boneless, skinless chicken breast, cut into ½-inch pieces

1 leek, green part only, chopped and washed (see headnote, page 110)

1 fennel bulb, chopped

1 cup chopped green beans

1 russet potato, cut into ½-inch cubes

5 cups Poultry Broth (page 195)

1 tablespoon cornstarch

1 teaspoon dried thyme

½ teaspoon sea salt

1. In a large pot, heat the oil over medium-high heat until it shimmers. Add the chicken, leek, and fennel and cook, stirring occasionally, until the chicken is cooked, about 5 minutes.

2. Add the green beans and potato.

3. In a small bowl, whisk together the broth and cornstarch. Add to the pot along with the thyme and salt. Cook, stirring occasionally, until the potatoes are soft, about 10 minutes more.

Serving size: 2 cups Calories: 179; Protein: 11g; Total fat: 5g; Saturated fat: 1g; Carbohydrates: 19g; Fiber: 4g; Sodium: 296mg

Easy Turkey Burgers

PREP TIME: 10 MINUTES; COOK TIME: 10 MINUTES

Fish sauce may seem like an odd add-in to a turkey burger, but it is the secret to flavor in this recipe; it adds a deep umami taste without even a hint of fishiness. The result is a wonderfully flavorful turkey burger. This is a great recipe to double or triple for a crowd.
SERVES 2

HEAL

REINTRODUCE

5-INGREDIENT
30-MINUTE

6 ounces ground
  turkey breast

½ teaspoon fish sauce

2 teaspoons sugar

½ teaspoon sea salt

1 tablespoon olive oil

2 gluten-free hamburger
  buns, toasted

4 tablespoons Burger
  Sauce (page 198)

1. In a medium bowl, combine the turkey breast, fish sauce, sugar, and salt. Mix well. Form into two patties.

2. In a large nonstick skillet, heat the oil over medium-high heat until it shimmers, swirling it to coat the pan.

3. Add the turkey burgers and cook until browned on both sides, 6 to 7 minutes total.

4. Spread each bun with 2 tablespoons of burger sauce, and top with the turkey burgers.

FLAVOR BOOST: Add a slice of Swiss cheese and a piece of lettuce.

SUBSTITUTION: For REINTRODUCE, add a slice of tomato to the burger.

Serving size: 1 burger Calories: 355; Protein: 25g; Total fat: 13g; Saturated fat: 2g; Carbohydrates: 38g; Fiber: 4g; Sodium: 955mg

Turkey Meatballs

PREP TIME: 10 MINUTES; COOK TIME: 20 MINUTES

Meatballs are great because they keep and reheat very well. You can freeze them in single portions and grab them for meals on the go. They'll keep for up to 3 days in the refrigerator or up to 6 months in the freezer. If you eat on the run a lot, double or triple the batch for less cooking in the future. SERVES 2

30-MINUTE

½ cup gluten-free bread crumbs

½ cup lactose-free nonfat milk

6 ounces ground turkey breast

¼ cup chopped fresh cilantro

1 tablespoon grated fresh ginger

1 teaspoon ground mustard

½ teaspoon sea salt

1. Preheat the oven to 375°F. Line a rimmed baking sheet with parchment paper or grease the baking sheet.

2. In a small bowl, combine the bread crumbs and milk, and let sit for 5 minutes.

3. In a medium bowl, combine the turkey breast, cilantro, ginger, mustard, salt, and bread crumb mixture. Combine well without overworking it (using your hands helps here).

4. Roll the mixture into 12 meatballs and place them on the prepared baking sheet.

5. Bake until the meatballs are cooked through, 15 to 20 minutes.

SUBSTITUTION: You can replace the ground turkey with extra-lean ground beef or ground chicken. For REINTRODUCE, add ½ garlic clove, minced, to the meat mixture.

Serving size: 6 meatballs Calories: 158; Protein: 24g; Total fat: 2g; Saturated fat: 0g; Carbohydrates: 12g; Fiber: 1g; Sodium: 592mg

STOP

HEAL

REINTRODUCE

Turkey Meatloaf Muffins

PREP TIME: 10 MINUTES; COOK TIME: 30 MINUTES

These simple meatloaf muffins take a while to cook, but it's all passive time. You can whip them together in about 10 minutes and enjoy your evening until they're ready to come out of the oven. You'll need a 6-muffin tin. Fill the remaining two muffin cups with a bit of water to keep them from burning. SERVES 4

5-INGREDIENT

Nonstick cooking spray

12 ounces ground turkey

¾ cup gluten-free
   bread crumbs

1 large egg, beaten

1 teaspoon Dijon mustard

1 tablespoon dried thyme

¾ teaspoon sea salt

1. Preheat the oven to 350°F. Coat a muffin tin with non-stick cooking spray.

2. In a medium bowl, combine all the ingredients.

3. Divide the mixture among four of the muffin cups. Bake until the internal temperature of the muffins is 165°F, about 20 minutes.

FLAVOR BOOST: Add ½ teaspoon fish sauce to the mixture.

SUBSTITUTE: For REINTRODUCE, add ½ onion, grated on a box grater.

Serving size: 1 muffin Calories: 136; Protein: 22g; Total fat: 3g; Saturated fat: 1g; Carbohydrates: 6g; Fiber: 1g; Sodium: 461mg

Turkey and Spinach Rollatini

PREP TIME: 10 MINUTES; COOK TIME: 25 MINUTES

Rolling turkey around a spinach and feta filling is a great way to get your meat and veggies in a simple meal. You'll need to soak the toothpicks before inserting them so they don't burn when they're in the oven. To pound the turkey, place it between two pieces of parchment paper and pound with a meat mallet or rolling pin. SERVES 4

5-INGREDIENT
ONE-PAN

12 ounces boneless,
   skinless turkey breast,
   pounded ¼ inch thick

½ teaspoon sea salt

1 cup frozen
   spinach, thawed

1 teaspoon grated
   lemon zest

¼ cup crumbled
   feta cheese

1. Preheat the oven to 325°F. Line a rimmed baking sheet with parchment paper or grease the baking sheet.

2. Place the turkey on the baking sheet, and sprinkle with the salt.

3. Spread the spinach over the turkey and sprinkle with the lemon zest and feta. Roll up the turkey around the filling and secure with either butcher's twine or pre-soaked toothpicks.

4. Bake until the internal temperature of the rollatini is 165°F, about 25 minutes. Cut crosswise into four sections to serve.

FLAVOR BOOST: For added texture, add ¼ cup pine nuts to the filling.

Serving size: ¼ recipe Calories: 214; Protein: 36g; Total fat: 5g; Saturated fat: 2g; Carbohydrates: 4g; Fiber: 1g; Sodium: 1208mg

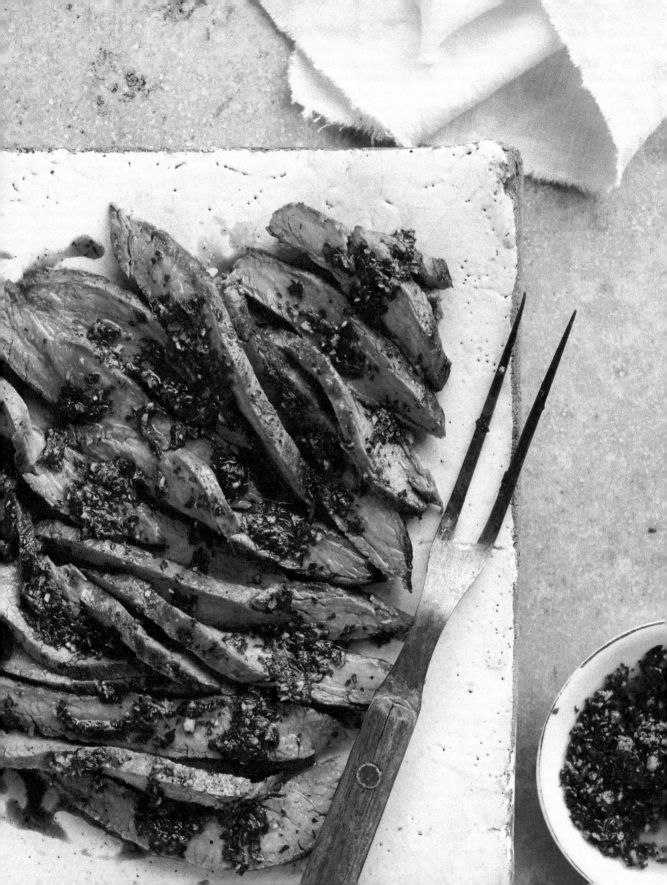

8
Beef and Lamb

Vegetable Beef Soup 154

Pho with Beef and
Zucchini Noodles 155

Patty Melt Soup 156

Sirloin Steak Salad with
Papaya Vinaigrette 157

Inside-Out Cabbage Rolls 158

Hamburger Stroganoff with
Zucchini Noodles 159

Hamburger Stew 160

Beef Tacos 161

Flank Steak with Chimichurri 162

Shepherd's Pie Muffins 163

Lamb Meatballs with
Lemon Yogurt Sauce 164

Ground Lamb and Lentil Chili 165

Herb-Crusted Lamb Chops 166

Roasted Lamb Chops with
Chimichurri 167

Lamb and Chickpea Stew 168

Open-Faced Stuffed Burgers 169

Flank Steak with Chimichurri, page 162

Vegetable Beef Soup

PREP TIME: 10 MINUTES; COOK TIME: 10 MINUTES

This soup will freeze and reheat well, so if you eat a lot of meals on the go, cook up a big batch. Freeze it in single-serving containers for up to 6 months, and reheat in the microwave as needed. SERVES 4

**30-MINUTE
ONE-PAN**

1 tablespoon olive oil

8 ounces extra-lean
  ground beef

1 leek, green part only,
  chopped and washed
  (see headnote, page 110)

1 carrot, peeled
  and chopped

1 fennel bulb, cored
  and chopped

1 cup halved green beans

7 cups Poultry Broth
  (page 195)

1 teaspoon dried thyme

½ teaspoon sea salt

1. In a large pot, heat the olive oil over medium-high heat until it shimmers. Add the ground beef, leek, carrot, and fennel and cook, stirring occasionally, until the beef is browned and the vegetables are tender, about 5 minutes.

2. Add the green beans, broth, thyme, and salt. Bring to a simmer, then reduce the heat to medium and simmer for 5 minutes.

SUBSTITUTION: If you can't find fennel, substitute 1 celery stalk and 1 zucchini, chopped. For REINTRODUCE, replace the leek with ½ onion, chopped.

Serving size: 2 cups Calories: 162; Protein: 13g; Total fat: 8g; Saturated fat: 2g; Carbohydrates: 11g; Fiber: 4g; Sodium: 316g

Pho with Beef and Zucchini Noodles

PREP TIME: 10 MINUTES; COOK TIME: 20 MINUTES

Even if you don't have a spiralizer, you can easily create zucchini noodles. Use a vegetable peeler to cut the zucchini lengthwise into long ribbons and then a paring knife to cut the ribbons into noodles. SERVES 4

30-MINUTE
ONE-PAN

8 cups Poultry Broth (page 195)

2 whole star anise

2 (1-inch) pieces peeled ginger

½ teaspoon sea salt

3 medium zucchini, cut into "spaghetti" noodles (see headnote)

8 ounces sirloin, cut into very thin (¼ inch or less) strips

¼ cup bean sprouts, for garnish

¼ cup chopped fresh cilantro, for garnish

Grated zest of 1 lime, for garnish

1. In a large pot, combine the broth, star anise, ginger, and salt. Simmer over medium-high heat for 15 minutes. Remove and discard the anise and ginger.

2. Divide the zucchini noodles among four bowls and top with the sirloin strips.

3. Pour the hot broth over the noodles. Allow the broth to cook the noodles and beef for 5 minutes.

4. Garnish with the bean sprouts, cilantro, and lime zest.

SUBSTITUTION: If you don't want to make the zucchini noodles, you may be able to find them premade in the produce section of the grocery store. Alternatively, you can use cooked gluten-free spaghetti (¼ to ½ cup per bowl). For REINTRODUCE, add ½ teaspoon garlic powder to the broth.

Serving size: 2 cups Calories: 161; Protein: 14g; Total fat: 8g; Saturated fat: 2g; Carbohydrates: 6g; Fiber: 2g; Sodium: 319g

STOP

HEAL

REINTRODUCE

Patty Melt Soup

PREP TIME: 10 MINUTES; COOK TIME: 15 MINUTES

The green part of a leek stands in here for caramelized onions, giving a hint of the flavor of a patty melt. Adding ground caraway seeds and mustard mimics the other flavors in the delicious sandwich. This soup will keep well, so it's an excellent choice for making ahead and freezing or refrigerating. SERVES 4

**30-MINUTE
ONE-PAN**

1 tablespoon unsalted grass-fed butter

8 ounces extra-lean ground beef

1 leek, green part only, finely chopped and washed (see headnote, page 110)

8 cups Poultry Broth (page 195)

1 teaspoon ground mustard

1 teaspoon ground caraway seeds

½ teaspoon sea salt

½ cup grated Cheddar cheese, for garnish

1. In a large pot, melt the butter over medium-high heat. Add the ground beef and leek. Cook, crumbling the beef with a spoon, until it is browned, 5 to 7 minutes.

2. Add the broth, mustard, caraway seeds, and salt. Bring to a simmer. Cook for 5 minutes more.

3. Serve garnished with the Cheddar.

SUBSTITUTION: If you can't find ground caraway, you can grind caraway seeds in a coffee or spice grinder. Alternatively, substitute 1 teaspoon ground cumin. For REINTRODUCE, omit the leek. Thinly slice ½ onion and cook it with the beef.

Serving size: 2 cups Calories: 197; Protein: 16g; Total fat: 11g; Saturated fat: 6g; Carbohydrates: 4g; Fiber: 1g; Sodium: 453g

Sirloin Steak Salad with Papaya Vinaigrette

PREP TIME: 10 MINUTES; COOK TIME: 10 MINUTES

If you're looking for a light and flavorful dinner salad for a warm night, you'll enjoy this recipe. The papaya vinaigrette adds a sweet, mellow flavor that pairs well with the thinly sliced sirloin steak. SERVES 2

5-INGREDIENT
30-MINUTE

1 teaspoon ground cumin

1 teaspoon dried oregano

½ teaspoon sea salt

4 ounces sirloin steak

1 tablespoon olive oil

4 cups torn
   romaine lettuce

4 tablespoons Papaya
   Vinaigrette (page 196)

1. In a small bowl, combine the cumin, oregano, and salt. Season the steak on both sides with the spice mixture.

2. In a large nonstick skillet, heat the oil over medium-high heat until it shimmers. Add the sirloin. Cook for about 5 minutes per side for medium-rare.

3. Slice the steak and toss with the lettuce and papaya vinaigrette.

SUBSTITUTION: To make this work for the HEAL plan, replace the vinaigrette with one of the other salad dressings in chapter 10.

Serving size: 2 ounces steak, 2 cups lettuce, 2 tablespoons vinaigrette Calories: 180; Protein: 13g; Total fat: 12g; Saturated fat: 2g; Carbohydrates: 8g; Fiber: 2g; Sodium: 731mg

STOP

REINTRODUCE

Inside-Out Cabbage Rolls

PREP TIME: 10 MINUTES; COOK TIME: 10 MINUTES

If you're a fan of cabbage rolls but don't want to spend the time it takes to roll and bake them, then try this quick stir-fry, which provides the same delicious flavors. While the recipe calls for napa cabbage, you can also use bok choy. Both are relatively low in acid.

SERVES 2

30-MINUTE
ONE-PAN

1 tablespoon olive oil

6 ounces extra-lean
ground beef

1 leek, green part only,
chopped and washed
(see headnote, page 110)

2 cups chopped
napa cabbage

1 teaspoon
ground mustard

1 teaspoon dried thyme

½ teaspoon sea salt

1 cup cooked brown rice

1. In a large nonstick skillet, heat the oil over medium-high heat until it shimmers.

2. Add the ground beef, leek, cabbage, mustard, thyme, and salt. Cook, crumbling the ground beef with a spoon, until it is browned, about 5 minutes.

3. Add the rice. Cook to heat it through, about 4 minutes more.

FLAVOR BOOST: If you're in REINTRODUCE, add ½ cup chopped fresh tomatoes when you add the rice.

Serving size: 2 cups Calories: 294; Protein: 22g; Total fat: 11g; Saturated fat: 4g; Carbohydrates: 25g; Fiber: 3g; Sodium: 577g

Hamburger Stroganoff with Zucchini Noodles

PREP TIME: 10 MINUTES; COOK TIME: 20 MINUTES

Using hamburger with classic stroganoff flavors makes this a quick, easy, and delicious meal. Use your vegetable peeler to cut the zucchini into ribbon noodles by peeling long strips lengthwise. SERVES 2

30-MINUTE

1 tablespoon olive oil

6 ounces extra-lean ground beef

1 cup sliced cremini mushrooms

1 leek, green part only, chopped and washed (see headnote, page 110)

1 teaspoon dried thyme

½ teaspoon sea salt

2 cups Poultry Broth (page 195)

1 cup lactose-free nonfat milk

1 tablespoon cornstarch

2 small zucchini, cut into ribbons (see headnote)

1. In a large nonstick skillet, heat the oil over medium-high heat until it shimmers.

2. Add the ground beef, mushrooms, leek, thyme, and salt. Cook, crumbling the ground beef with a spoon, until it is browned, about 5 minutes.

3. In a small bowl, whisk together the broth, milk, and cornstarch. Add to the skillet along with the zucchini noodles and cook, stirring, until the sauce thickens slightly, about 2 minutes.

FLAVOR BOOST: Garnish the dish with ¼ cup chopped fresh parsley.

Serving size: 2 cups Calories: 291; Protein: 25g; Total fat: 10g; Saturated fat: 2g; Carbohydrates: 22g; Fiber: 3g; Sodium: 592g

Hamburger Stew

PREP TIME: 10 MINUTES; COOK TIME: 15 MINUTES

Traditional beef stew takes a while to cook because stew meat needs a few hours of braising to get tender. Using ground beef shortens the time and yields a flavorful stew that's a perfect winter meal. This keeps well in the freezer, so it's a good make-ahead meal. SERVES 4

30-MINUTE
ONE-PAN

1 tablespoon olive oil

9 ounces extra-lean
  ground beef

1 leek, green part only,
  chopped and washed
  (see headnote, page 110)

2 carrots, peeled
  and chopped

1 cup corn kernels, fresh
  or frozen

1 russet potato,
  peeled and cut into
  ½-inch cubes

4 cups Poultry Broth
  (page 195)

1 tablespoon cornstarch

1 teaspoon dried thyme

½ teaspoon sea salt

1. In a large pot, heat the oil over medium-high heat until it shimmers.

2. Add the ground beef and leek. Cook, crumbling the ground beef with a spoon, until it is browned, about 5 minutes.

3. Add the carrots, corn, and potato.

4. Whisk together the broth, cornstarch, thyme, and salt. Add to the stew.

5. Cook, stirring occasionally, until the potatoes are tender, about 10 minutes.

FLAVOR BOOST: Add 1 teaspoon ground mustard to the broth before adding it to the stew.

SUBSTITUTION: For REINTRODUCE, replace the leek with ½ onion, chopped.

Serving size: 2 cups Calories: 173; Protein: 14g; Total fat: 6g; Saturated fat: 3g; Carbohydrates: 16g; Fiber: 2g; Sodium: 266g

Beef Tacos

PREP TIME: 10 MINUTES; COOK TIME: 15 MINUTES

What's a week without taco night? These beef tacos are quick and easy, and if you store the components separately, they travel well. Make up a batch of beef and store it in single-serving containers, then take all the other ingredients with you for tacos on the go.

SERVES 4

30-MINUTE

4 corn tortillas

1 tablespoon olive oil

9 ounces extra-lean ground beef

1 leek, green part only, chopped and washed (see headnote, page 110)

1 teaspoon ground cumin

1 teaspoon ground coriander

½ teaspoon sea salt

½ avocado, chopped

½ cup grated Cheddar cheese

¼ cup Yogurt Sour Cream (page 208)

1. Preheat the oven to 350°F. Wrap the tortillas in aluminum foil and heat in the oven for 15 minutes.

2. Meanwhile, in a large nonstick skillet, heat the oil over medium-high heat until it shimmers.

3. Add the ground beef, leek, cumin, coriander, and salt. Cook, crumbling the ground beef with a spoon, until it is browned, about 5 minutes.

4. To assemble the tacos, portion the beef on the tortillas. Top with the avocado, Cheddar, and sour cream.

FLAVOR BOOST: Garnish the tacos with ¼ cup chopped fresh cilantro and 1 teaspoon grated lime zest.

SUBSTITUTION: For REINTRODUCE, add ½ green bell pepper, finely chopped, to the beef, or replace the leek with ½ onion, chopped.

Serving size: 1 taco Calories: 298; Protein: 19g; Total fat: 16g; Saturated fat: 7g; Carbohydrates: 18g; Fiber: 4g; Sodium: 503mg

HEAL

REINTRODUCE

Flank Steak with Chimichurri

PREP TIME: 10 MINUTES; COOK TIME: 10 MINUTES

Flank steak cooks quickly on the stove top or grill, and it's a cut of meat that has a lot of flavor. Slicing it against the grain helps tenderize it. The chimichurri sauce adds loads of flavor. SERVES 4

30-MINUTE

1 teaspoon dried oregano

1 teaspoon ground cumin

½ teaspoon sea
  salt, divided

1 (12-ounce) flank steak

3 tablespoons olive
  oil, divided

½ cup chopped
  fresh parsley

¼ cup chopped fresh
  cilantro

Grated zest of ½ lime

1. In a small bowl, stir together the oregano, cumin, and ¼ teaspoon of salt. Sprinkle evenly over the flank steak.

2. Heat 1 tablespoon of oil in a large nonstick skillet over medium-high heat until it shimmers.

3. Add the flank steak and cook for 2 to 3 minutes per side.

4. Reduce the heat to low. Continue cooking until the steak it reaches 135°F for medium-rare, about 5 minutes more.

5. Meanwhile, in a blender or food processor, combine the remaining 2 tablespoons of oil, parsley, cilantro, lime zest, and remaining ¼ teaspoon of sea salt. Pulse 20 times, or until it is well combined.

6. Slice the flank steak thinly slices against the grain. Serve with the chimichurri.

SUBSTITUTION: For REINTRODUCE, add ½ garlic clove, minced, to the blender or food processor for the chimichurri.

Serving size: 3 ounces steak, 2 tablespoons chimichurri
Calories: 276; Protein: 24g; Total fat: 20g; Saturated fat: 6g; Carbohydrates: 1g; Fiber: <1g; Sodium: 310mg

Shepherd's Pie Muffins

PREP TIME: 10 MINUTES; COOK TIME: 10 MINUTES

With a traditional shepherd's pie, baking takes about an hour. Here we speed it up by cooking the filling on the stove top, spooning the mashed potatoes on top, and broiling it briefly to melt the cheese. It makes a quick and tasty hearty meal. SERVES 3

30-MINUTE

6 ounces ground lamb

1 leek, green part only, chopped and washed (see headnote, page 110)

1 carrot, peeled and chopped

1 cup green peas

1 teaspoon dried thyme

½ teaspoon sea salt

1 recipe Mashed Potatoes (page 101)

½ cup grated Cheddar cheese

1. Preheat the broiler on high.

2. Heat a large nonstick skillet over medium-high heat.

3. Combine the ground lamb, leek, carrot, peas, thyme, and salt in the skillet. Cook, crumbling the lamb with a spoon, until the vegetables are soft and the lamb is cooked, 5 to 7 minutes.

4. Divide the meat mixture evenly among four cups in a muffin tin. Top each muffin with mashed potatoes and sprinkle Cheddar over the top.

5. Broil until the cheese melts, about 3 minutes.

SUBSTITUTION: To make this suitable for HEAL, replace the peas with ½ cup corn. For REINTRODUCE, replace the leek with ½ small onion, finely chopped.

Serving size: 2 muffins Calories: 361; Protein: 21g; Total fat: 24g; Saturated fat: 13g; Carbohydrates: 42g; Fiber: 5g; Sodium: 886g

Lamb Meatballs with Lemon Yogurt Sauce

PREP TIME: 10 MINUTES; COOK TIME: 20 MINUTES

Made with tasty Mediterranean spices, these meatballs are aromatic, flavorful, quick, and easy. Serve them with brown rice and a steamed vegetable or salad for a full meal.

SERVES 2

5-INGREDIENT
30-MINUTE

Nonstick cooking spray

6 ounces ground lamb

½ teaspoon ground cinnamon

½ teaspoon ground cumin

½ teaspoon ground allspice

½ teaspoon sea salt

¼ cup Lemon Yogurt Sauce (page 199)

1. Preheat the oven to 400°F. Coat a rimmed baking sheet with nonstick cooking spray.

2. In a bowl, combine the ground lamb with the cinnamon, cumin, allspice, and salt.

3. Roll the mixture into 12 meatballs and place them on the prepared baking sheet.

4. Bake until the lamb reaches an internal temperature of 145°F, about 20 minutes.

5. Serve with the yogurt sauce for dipping.

FLAVOR BOOST: Whisk 1 tablespoon tahini into the lemon yogurt sauce and add ¼ cup chopped fresh parsley.

SUBSTITUTION: For REINTRODUCE, add ½ garlic clove, minced, to the lamb mixture.

Serving size: 6 meatballs Calories: 242; Protein: 16g; Total fat: 11g; Saturated fat: 6g; Carbohydrates: 1g; Fiber: 1g; Sodium: 518g

Ground Lamb and Lentil Chili

PREP TIME: 10 MINUTES; COOK TIME: 10 MINUTES

Typically, ground lamb isn't considered a candidate for chili, but it works here with the spice profile. This freezes well for up to 6 months, so you can make a larger batch and portion it into single servings, then freeze it for when you need a tasty meal in a hurry.

SERVES 4

30-MINUTE
ONE-PAN

12 ounces ground lamb

1 leek, green part only, chopped and washed (see headnote, page 110)

2 cups canned lentils

1 cup Poultry Broth (page 195)

1 tablespoon ground cumin

1 teaspoon ground coriander

½ teaspoon sea salt

1 teaspoon grated lime zest, for garnish

¼ cup chopped fresh cilantro, for garnish

1. Heat a large pot over medium-high heat. Cook the ground lamb and leek, crumbling the meat with a spoon, until it is browned, about 5 minutes.

2. Add the lentils, broth, cumin, coriander, and salt. Cook, stirring occasionally, for 5 more minutes.

3. Garnish with the lime zest and cilantro.

FLAVOR BOOST: Garnish each bowl of chili with ⅛ avocado, chopped.

SUBSTITUTION: For REINTRODUCE, replace the leek with ½ small onion, finely chopped; or add ½ tomato, chopped, when you add the lentils.

Serving size: 2 cups Calories: 317; Protein: 21g; Total fat: 11g; Saturated fat: 6g; Carbohydrates: 17g; Fiber: 4g; Sodium: 465g

Herb-Crusted Lamb Chops

PREP TIME: 10 MINUTES; COOK TIME: 10 MINUTES

This recipe uses lamb loin chops, which are smaller and more tender than a typical lamb chop. The herb crust is easy to make in your food processor or blender; you'll need gluten-free bread crumbs and lots of herbs, but it makes the lamb incredibly flavorful.

SERVES 2

30-MINUTE

¾ cup gluten-free bread crumbs

1 tablespoon unsalted grass-fed butter, at room temperature

1 teaspoon Dijon mustard

¼ cup fresh rosemary leaves

¼ cup fresh oregano leaves

¼ cup fresh parsley

½ teaspoon sea salt

4 lamb loin chops

1 tablespoon olive oil

1. Preheat the oven to 325°F.

2. In a blender or food processor, pulse the bread crumbs, butter, mustard, rosemary, oregano, parsley, and salt 20 times, or until the herbs are chopped and well combined with the bread crumbs.

3. Spread the mixture on the lamb chops, pressing so it sticks to the surface of the meat.

4. In a large nonstick skillet, heat the olive oil over medium-high heat until it shimmers.

5. Add the chops. Brown them for 3 minutes per side, then transfer to a rimmed baking sheet.

6. Bake for 6 minutes, or until the lamb reaches an internal temperature of 145°F.

SUBSTITUTION: If you can't find fresh oregano (which is typically the most difficult of these herbs to find), substitute 2 teaspoons dried oregano. For REINTRODUCE, add ½ garlic clove, minced, to the herb mixture.

Serving size: 2 chops Calories: 485; Protein: 21g; Total fat: 40g; Saturated fat: 16g; Carbohydrates: 10g; Fiber: 2g; Sodium: 664g

Roasted Lamb Chops with Chimichurri

PREP TIME: 10 MINUTES; COOK TIME: 15 MINUTES

A quick sear and roast of seasoned lamb loin chops is all the cooking required for these tasty chops. The sauce, which is quick and easy to make, adds lots of flavor. SERVES 2

5-INGREDIENT
30-MINUTE

4 lamb loin chops

½ teaspoon sea salt

1 tablespoon olive oil

½ cup Oregano and Parsley Chimichurri (page 205)

1. Preheat the oven to 325°F.

2. Season the lamb chops with the salt.

3. In a large nonstick skillet, heat the oil over medium-high heat until it shimmers.

4. Add the chops. Brown them for 3 minutes per side, then transfer to a rimmed baking sheet.

5. Bake for 6 minutes, or until the lamb reaches an internal temperature of 145°F.

6. Serve with the chimichurri spooned over the top.

FLAVOR BOOST: Add 1 teaspoon dried oregano and ½ teaspoon ground cumin to the salt and sprinkle it on the chops before searing them.

Serving size: 2 chops Calories: 421; Protein: 46; Total fat: 25g; Saturated fat: 6g; Carbohydrates: 2g; Fiber: <1g; Sodium: 975g

Lamb and Chickpea Stew

PREP TIME: 10 MINUTES; COOK TIME: 10 MINUTES

This fragrant stew has aromatic spices that will leave your kitchen smelling divine. It freezes well, so cook up a larger batch if you'd like a freezer full of meals ready to go.

SERVES 4

30-MINUTE

9 ounces ground lamb

1 leek, green part only, chopped and washed (see headnote, page 110)

1 cup canned chickpeas

1 teaspoon grated orange zest

1 teaspoon ground cumin

½ teaspoon ground allspice

½ teaspoon ground cinnamon

½ teaspoon sea salt

2 cups Poultry Broth (page 195)

1 tablespoon cornstarch

1. Heat a large pot over medium-high heat. Cook the ground lamb and leek, crumbling the meat with a spoon until it is browned, about 5 minutes.

2. Add the chickpeas, orange zest, cumin, allspice, cinnamon, and salt.

3. In a small bowl, whisk together the broth and cornstarch, then add it to the stew.

4. Bring to a boil and lower the heat to medium. Simmer for 5 minutes.

FLAVOR BOOST: Add 1 cup stemmed and chopped kale or Swiss chard when you add the lamb and leek.

SUBSTITUTION: For REINTRODUCE, you can replace the leek with ½ small onion, chopped.

Serving size: 2 cups Calories: 208; Protein: 13g; Total fat: 9g; Saturated fat: 5g; Carbohydrates: 8g; Fiber: 2g; Sodium: 359mg

Open-Faced Stuffed Burgers

PREP TIME: 10 MINUTES; COOK TIME: 15 MINUTES

Adding herbs and cheese to the inside of a burger makes it seem moister, which is a nice trick when you're using low-fat meat. This recipe also uses a panade, which is a bread-based paste that will help the meat retain moisture. The burger sauce adds a surprising final burst of flavor to this open-faced sandwich. SERVES 4

½ cup lactose-free
  nonfat milk

¼ cup gluten-free
  bread crumbs

1 pound extra-lean
  ground beef

½ teaspoon sea salt

1 teaspoon Dijon mustard

½ teaspoon fish sauce

½ cup grated
  Cheddar cheese

4 tablespoons finely
  chopped, fresh basil

4 slices gluten-free
  bread, toasted

4 tablespoons Burger
  Sauce (page 198)

1. In a small bowl, combine the milk and bread crumbs. Allow to rest for 10 minutes.

2. In a medium bowl, combine the ground beef, bread crumb mixture, salt, mustard, and fish sauce until well mixed. Roll into eight balls and pat each out into a ¼-inch thick patty.

3. In a small bowl, mix the cheese and basil. Sprinkle the cheese mixture on each of four patties and top with another patty. Pinch the edges to seal.

4. Preheat a nonstick skillet on medium-high. Place the burger patties in the skillet and heat until cooked, about 5 minutes per side.

5. Serve on the toasted bread with 1 tablespoon of the Burger Sauce spooned over the top of each.

SUBSTITUTION TIP: For REINTRODUCE, add 1 finely minced garlic clove to the ground beef mixture.

Serving size: 1 patty, 1 slice bread Calories: 366; Protein: 30g; Total fat: 17g; Saturated Fat: 9g; Carbohydrates: 24g; Fiber: 1g; Sodium: 803mg

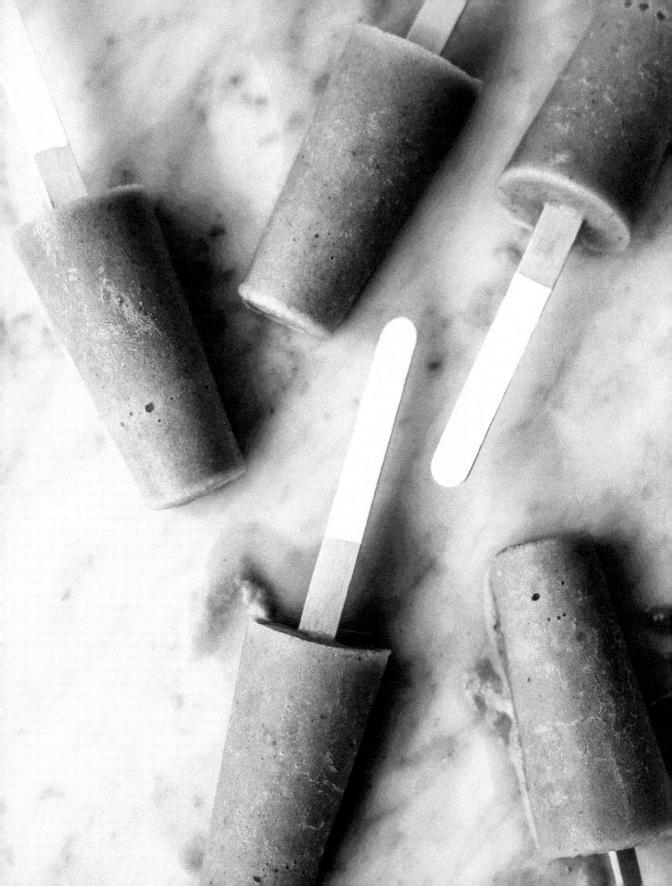

9

Snacks and Sweets

Deviled Eggs 172

Spiced Walnuts 173

Cinnamon-Sugar Popcorn 174

Cucumber Rounds with
    Shrimp Salad 175

Baked Potato Chips 176

Carrots with Herbed
    Yogurt Dip 177

Turkey-Wrapped Melon 178

Grated Carrot and Raisin Salad 179

Peanut Butter and Carob Balls 180

Peanut Butter and Banana
    Spread with Ginger 181

Melon with Ginger
    Dipping Sauce 182

Melon Granita 183

Honeydew and Cilantro
    Ice Pops 184

Yogurt and Melon Ice Pops 185

Brûléed Bananas 186

Banana Ice Cream 187

Banana and Melon Salad 188

Almond Meringue Cookies 189

Peanut Butter Cookies 190

Banana Pudding 191

Honeydew and Cilantro Ice Pops, page 184

Deviled Eggs

PREP TIME: 10 MINUTES; COOK TIME: 14 MINUTES

Deviled eggs make a great take-it-and-go snack. They'll keep in the refrigerator for up to 3 days. They're also a great choice for a party appetizer if you want to make a big batch to share with family and friends. Eggs that are slightly less fresh are easier to peel. SERVES 4

5-INGREDIENT

30-MINUTE

4 large eggs

¼ cup lactose-free nonfat plain yogurt

1 teaspoon Dijon mustard

1 tablespoon chopped fresh dill

¼ teaspoon sea salt

1. Put the eggs in a medium saucepan and cover with water by at least 1 inch.

2. Bring the water to a boil over medium-high heat, then immediately remove the pot from the heat, cover with a lid, and allow the eggs to sit in the hot water for 14 minutes.

3. Under running water, peel the eggs. Slice them in half lengthwise and gently spoon out the yolks. Put the yolks in a small bowl and arrange the whites on a plate with the cut side up.

4. Add the yogurt, mustard, dill, and salt to the yolks. Blend with a fork until smooth. Spoon the yolk mixture back into the egg halves.

FLAVOR BOOST: Add 2 tablespoons chopped fresh basil to the yolk mixture and ½ teaspoon grated lemon zest.

Serving size: 1 egg Calories: 84; Protein: 7g; Total fat: 5g; Saturated fat: 2g; Carbohydrates: 2g; Fiber: <1g; Sodium: 205mg

Spiced Walnuts

PREP TIME: 5 MINUTES; COOK TIME: 5 MINUTES

These walnuts will keep well for up to a week in a resealable bag or airtight container. They're delicious as a snack, or you can toss them on a salad or with some melons and bananas for a crunchy, sweet snack or dessert. SERVES 4

5-INGREDIENT
30-MINUTE
ONE-PAN

2 tablespoons unsalted grass-fed butter

¼ cup dark brown sugar

½ teaspoon ground ginger

¼ teaspoon ground cloves

24 walnuts, shelled

1. In a medium nonstick skillet, melt the butter over medium-high heat.

2. Add the brown sugar, ginger, and cloves. Cook, stirring, until it boils.

3. Add the walnuts and cook, stirring, for 3 minutes.

4. Cool before serving.

FLAVOR BOOST: Add ½ teaspoon grated orange zest to the spice mixture.

Serving size: 6 walnuts Calories: 183; Protein: 4g;
Total fat: 15g; Saturated fat: 4g; Carbohydrates: 11g; Fiber: 1g;
Sodium: 44mg

STOP

HEAL

REINTRODUCE

Cinnamon-Sugar Popcorn

PREP TIME: 5 MINUTES

Air-popped popcorn is good plain, but when you add butter, cinnamon, and sugar, it goes from a workaday snack to something really tasty. Plus, it's easy to make—it takes only a few minutes, and you can make it anytime you wish. SERVES 2

5-INGREDIENT

30-MINUTE

¼ cup sugar

1 teaspoon ground cinnamon

6 cups air-popped popcorn

2 tablespoons unsalted grass-fed butter, melted

1. In a small bowl, combine the sugar and cinnamon.

2. In a large bowl, toss the cinnamon-sugar with the popcorn and butter.

FLAVOR BOOST: Add ¼ teaspoon ground cardamom to the spice mix.

Serving size 3 cups Calories: 290; Protein: 3g; Total fat: 12g; Saturated fat: 7g; Carbohydrates: 46g; Fiber: 4g; Sodium: 6mg

Cucumber Rounds with Shrimp Salad

PREP TIME: 5 MINUTES

Orange zest and fresh tarragon bring out the sweetness of the shrimp in this salad, and cucumber rounds serve as a flavorful textural element, giving the dish a nice crisp crunch. This is an easy dish to take with you—carry the shrimp salad and cucumber rounds separately and put them together just before serving. SERVES 2

5-INGREDIENT
30-MINUTE
ONE-PAN

½ cup cooked
baby shrimp

2 tablespoons lactose-
free nonfat plain yogurt

1 tablespoon chopped
fresh tarragon

½ teaspoon grated
orange zest

1 medium
cucumber, sliced

1. In a small bowl, combine the shrimp with the yogurt, tarragon, and orange zest. Mix well.

2. Spoon the shrimp salad onto the cucumber rounds.

SUBSTITUTION: If you can't find fresh tarragon, substitute 1 tablespoon chopped fresh dill and replace the orange zest with an equal amount of lemon zest.

Calories: 63; Protein: 8g; Total fat: 1g; Saturated fat: <1g; Carbohydrates: 7g; Fiber: <1g; Sodium: 264mg

HEAL

REINTRODUCE

Baked Potato Chips

PREP TIME: 10 MINUTES; COOK TIME: 15 MINUTES

Served alone, these make a great snack. Alongside a sandwich, they're perfect for lunch. Or with a burger, you've got a quick side for your dinner. Regardless of how you serve them, these lightly salty potato chips will soothe your craving for crunchiness. SERVES 2

5-INGREDIENT

30-MINUTE

1 medium Yukon Gold
potato, cut into ⅛-inch-
thick slices

1 tablespoon olive oil

¼ to ½ teaspoon sea salt

1. Preheat the oven to 400°F.

2. In a large bowl, toss the potato slices with the olive oil and salt.

3. Spread the slices in a single layer on a rimmed baking sheet.

4. Bake until crisp, 12 to 15 minutes.

FLAVOR BOOST: Add 1 tablespoon chopped fresh rosemary when you toss the potatoes with the olive oil and salt.

Serving size: ½ batch Calories: 142; Protein: 2g; Total fat: 7g; Saturated fat: 1g; Carbohydrates: 19g; Fiber: 2g; Sodium: 474mg

Carrots with Herbed Yogurt Dip

PREP TIME: 10 MINUTES

This dip is great on carrots, but it's equally tasty on Baked Potato Chips (page 176) or with homemade Sweet Potato French Fries (page 96). It will keep for up to 5 days in the refrigerator, and the flavors actually blend a bit better the longer you keep it. SERVES 2

30-MINUTE

ONE-PAN

½ cup lactose-free nonfat plain yogurt

1 tablespoon chopped fresh dill

1 tablespoon chopped fresh thyme

1 tablespoon chopped fresh parsley

½ teaspoon grated lemon zest

¼ teaspoon sea salt

2 carrots, peeled and cut into sticks

1. In a small bowl, combine the yogurt, dill, thyme, parsley, lemon zest, and salt. Mix well.

2. Serve with the carrot sticks for dipping.

FLAVOR BOOST: Instead of the lemon zest and herbs listed here, add ½ teaspoon grated lime zest, 1 tablespoon chopped fresh cilantro, ½ teaspoon ground cumin, and ¼ teaspoon sea salt to the yogurt.

SUBSTITUTION: For REINTRODUCE, add ½ garlic clove, minced, to this dip.

Serving size: 1 carrot, ¼ cup dip Calories: 60; Protein: 4g; Total fat: <1g; Saturated fat: <1g; Carbohydrates: 11g; Fiber: 2g; Sodium: 327mg

HEAL

REINTRODUCE

Turkey-Wrapped Melon

PREP TIME: 5 MINUTES

This snack travels well, and you can put it together quickly if you have the ingredients on hand. If you're on the STOP plan, drizzle the melon with a little honey for added sweetness in place of the maple syrup. SERVES 2

5-INGREDIENT
30-MINUTE
ONE-PAN

8 (½-inch-thick)
honeydew wedges,
rind removed

1 tablespoon pure
maple syrup

1 tablespoon chopped
fresh tarragon

½ teaspoon grated
orange zest

8 slices deli turkey

1. In a large bowl, toss the melon wedges with the syrup, tarragon, and orange zest.

2. Place each wedge on a slice of deli turkey and wrap the turkey around the melon. Secure with a toothpick.

SUBSTITUTION: You can trade the honeydew for any seasonal melon (except watermelon), such as cantaloupe or casaba.

Serving size: 4 pieces Calories: 197; Protein: 15g; Total fat: 2g; Saturated fat: <1g; Carbohydrates: 34g; Fiber: 2g; Sodium: 906mg

Grated Carrot and Raisin Salad

This is a great side dish or snack. Or put it on Easy Turkey Burgers (page 148) for an extra hint of sweetness and crunch. When they're in season, substitute different colored carrots, such as purple, red, and white, to make the salad even more colorful. SERVES 2

5-INGREDIENT
30-MINUTE
ONE-PAN

3 carrots, peeled and grated on a box grater

¼ cup raisins

2 tablespoons lactose-free nonfat plain yogurt

1 tablespoon pure maple syrup

¼ teaspoon ground cinnamon

In a large bowl, mix all the ingredients until well combined.

SUBSTITUTION: To make this work for STOP, omit the raisins.

Serving size: ¼ cup Calories: 125; Protein: 2g; Total fat: <1g; Saturated fat: <1g; Carbohydrates: 32g; Fiber: 3g; Sodium: 76mg

HEAL

REINTRODUCE

Peanut Butter and Carob Balls

PREP TIME: 10 MINUTES

These satisfying treats keep well. Stick them in the refrigerator in a sealed container for up to a week. They contain protein for energy and aren't very high in sugar. If you can't find carob powder at your local grocery or health food store, it is available online.

MAKES 6

HEAL

REINTRODUCE

5-INGREDIENT

30-MINUTE

ONE-PAN

6 tablespoons crunchy peanut butter

3 tablespoons confectioners' sugar

1 tablespoon unsweetened carob powder

Pinch salt

1. In a medium bowl, mix all the ingredients until well combined.

2. Roll the mixture into 6 balls.

FLAVOR BOOST: For extra crunch, roll each ball in chopped peanuts.

Serving size: 1 ball Calories: 118; Protein: 4g; Total fat: 8g; Saturated fat: 2g; Carbohydrates: 9g; Fiber: 1g; Sodium: 102mg

Peanut Butter and Banana Spread with Ginger

PREP TIME: 10 MINUTES

Use this spread with carrots, celery, or gluten-free crackers. It keeps for up to 3 days in the refrigerator and travels well for snacks on the go. It's also super quick and easy to make if you're craving something a little sweet. SERVES 4

5-INGREDIENT
30-MINUTE
ONE-PAN

¼ cup peanut butter

½ banana, mashed

1 tablespoon pure
maple syrup

1 teaspoon grated
fresh ginger

Pinch salt

In a blender or food processor, mix all the ingredients until well combined.

FLAVOR BOOST: Add 1 tablespoon unsweetened carob powder.

Serving size: 2 tablespoons Calories: 123; Protein: 4g; Total fat: 8; Saturated fat: 2g; Carbohydrates: 10g; Fiber: 1g; Sodium: 42mg

STOP

HEAL

REINTRODUCE

Melon with Ginger Dipping Sauce

PREP TIME: 10 MINUTES

This recipe makes a lovely light, fresh dessert or a tasty snack. You can also combine the melon and sauce to make fruit salad, if you prefer. To serve to guests, use wooden skewers to create individual portions of melon. SERVES 4

5-INGREDIENT

30-MINUTE

ONE-PAN

1 cup lactose-free nonfat
   plain yogurt

1 tablespoon pure
   maple syrup

1 teaspoon grated
   fresh ginger

1 cup honeydew balls

1 cup cantaloupe balls

1. In a small bowl, whisk together the yogurt, syrup, and ginger.

2. Serve with the melon balls for dipping.

FLAVOR BOOST: Add ½ teaspoon grated orange zest and ½ teaspoon ground cinnamon to the yogurt along with the maple syrup and ginger.

Serving size: ½ cup melon, ¼ cup sauce Calories: 89; Protein: 4g; Total fat: <1; Saturated fat: <1g; Carbohydrates: 16g; Fiber: <1g; Sodium: 59mg

Melon Granita

PREP TIME: 10 MINUTES

The nice thing about this dessert is you can make the melon balls when you have a bit of time, and keep them in one-cup servings in the freezer for up to 3 months. You can then whip them out anytime you want to make this frozen sweet treat. SERVES 2

5-INGREDIENT
30-MINUTE
ONE-PAN

1 cup honeydew
   balls, frozen

1 cup cantaloupe
   balls, frozen

1 tablespoon pure
   maple syrup

1 teaspoon grated
   fresh ginger

In a blender or food processor, combine the melon balls, syrup, and ginger. Pulse 10 times. Serve immediately.

FLAVOR BOOST: Add ¼ teaspoon ground cardamom.

Serving size: ¼ cup Calories: 86; Protein: 1g; Total fat: <1; Saturated fat: <1g; Carbohydrates: 21g; Fiber: 2g; Sodium: 29mg

Honeydew and Cilantro Ice Pops

PREP TIME: 10 MINUTES (PLUS FREEZING TIME)

Honeydew and cilantro may seem like an odd combo for an ice pop, but with some lime zest in it as well, it's a refreshing, stevia-sweetened treat that's pretty tasty. SERVES 4

5-INGREDIENT

2 cups honeydew balls

1 cup lactose-free nonfat plain yogurt

¼ cup chopped fresh cilantro

Grated zest of 1 lime

2 packets stevia

1. In a blender or food processor, combine all the ingredients and process until smooth.

2. Pour into four ice pop molds. Freeze for at least 8 hours.

SUBSTITUTION: For REINTRODUCE, replace the stevia with 2 tablespoons honey.

Serving size: 1 pop Calories: 60; Protein: 3g; Total fat: <1; Saturated fat: <1g; Carbohydrates: 12g; Fiber: <1g; Sodium: 56mg

Yogurt and Melon Ice Pops

PREP TIME: 10 MINUTES (PLUS FREEZING TIME)

If you don't have ice pop molds, you can use paper cups instead. Just pour the mixture into the paper cups, cover them with aluminum foil, and poke an ice pop stick through the foil to hold it in place. Freeze, then peel away the paper cup to eat. SERVES 4

5-INGREDIENT

2 cups honeydew balls

1 cup lactose-free nonfat plain yogurt

2 tablespoons pure maple syrup

1. In a blender or food processor, combine all the ingredients and process until smooth.

2. Pour into four ice pop molds. Freeze for at least 8 hours.

SUBSTITUTION: Replace the honeydew with cantaloupe or another seasonal melon (except for watermelon). For REINTRODUCE, replace 1 cup of the melon balls with 1 cup hulled and sliced strawberries.

Serving size: 1 pop Calories: 100; Protein: 4g; Total fat: <1; Saturated fat: <1g; Carbohydrates: 18g; Fiber: <1g; Sodium: 59mg

HEAL

REINTRODUCE

Brûléed Bananas

PREP TIME: 10 MINUTES; COOK TIME: 5 MINUTES

"Brûlée" refers to the process of caramelizing sugar, which gives it a toasty flavor and a satisfying caramel crunch. If you have a kitchen blowtorch, you can use that to brûlée the sugar instead of the broiler. Eat these bananas by themselves, use them to top Banana Pudding (page 191), or serve them with ¼ cup of lactose-free plain yogurt combined with 1 tablespoon of maple syrup. SERVES 2

5-INGREDIENT
30-MINUTE
ONE-PAN

1 banana

3 tablespoons sugar

1. Preheat the broiler on high.

2. Peel the banana and cut it in half horizontally. Cut each half in half lengthwise. Place the pieces on a rimmed baking sheet, cut side up.

3. Sprinkle the bananas with the sugar. Place under the broiler until the sugar starts to melt and brown, 4 to 5 minutes. Check frequently to make sure they don't burn.

FLAVOR BOOST: Mix the sugar with ¼ teaspoon ground cinnamon before sprinkling on the banana.

Serving size: ½ banana Calories: 120; Protein: <1g; Total fat: <1; Saturated fat: <1g; Carbohydrates: 32g; Fiber: 2g; Sodium: 1mg

Banana Ice Cream

PREP TIME: 10 MINUTES

It doesn't get any easier than this banana ice cream. All you need to do is freeze the peeled bananas ahead of time—they'll be good for up to 6 months. Then just pull out the bananas when you're ready for a creamy, sweet treat. SERVES 2

5-INGREDIENT
30-MINUTE
ONE-PAN

2 bananas, peeled and frozen

1 tablespoon pure maple syrup

Pinch nutmeg

Combine all the ingredients in a food processor and blend until smooth.

FLAVOR BOOST: Sprinkle with chopped Spiced Walnuts (page 173).

Serving size: ½ recipe Calories: 132; Protein: 1g; Total fat: <1; Saturated fat: <1g; Carbohydrates: 34g; Fiber: 3g; Sodium: 2mg

Banana and Melon Salad

PREP TIME: 10 MINUTES

This simple fruit salad is sweet and satisfying as a snack, dessert, or side dish. Plus, it's easy to make; if you buy premade melon balls from the salad bar or produce section at the grocery store, it can be ready in less than 5 minutes. SERVES 4

5-INGREDIENT
30-MINUTE
ONE-PAN

2 bananas, peeled
   and sliced

2 cups cantaloupe balls

1 tablespoon pure
   maple syrup

¼ teaspoon grated
   orange zest

In a large bowl, mix all the ingredients until well combined.

FLAVOR BOOST: For REINTRODUCE, add ¼ cup shredded toasted coconut for texture and flavor.

SUBSTITUTION: For REINTRODUCE, add ½ cup blueberries.

Serving size: 1 cup Calories: 92; Protein: 1g; Total fat: <1; Saturated fat: <1g; Carbohydrates: 23g; Fiber: 2g; Sodium: 14mg

Almond Meringue Cookies

PREP TIME: 10 MINUTES; COOK TIME: 25 MINUTES

These cookies will keep for at least a week in an airtight container or resealable bag. The baking time is a bit long, but it results in a crisp, light cookie. Feel free to substitute vanilla for the almond extract if you're looking for a different flavor profile. For best results, beat the egg whites at room temperature and make sure they are entirely free of any bits of yolk, as fat keeps meringue from forming. MAKES 12

5-INGREDIENT

2 large egg whites

1 teaspoon almond extract

¼ teaspoon grated orange zest

⅛ teaspoon cream of tartar

Pinch salt

¾ cup sugar

1. Preheat the oven to 300°F. Line a baking sheet with parchment paper or grease the baking sheet.

2. In a large bowl, use an electric mixer to beat the egg whites, almond extract, orange zest, cream of tartar, and salt on high until the mixture forms stiff peaks.

3. With the mixer running, add the sugar in a thin stream until incorporated.

4. Spoon the meringue into 12 mounds on the prepared baking sheet.

5. Bake until crisped and slightly browned, about 25 minutes.

SUBSTITUTION: Substitute maple sugar for the white sugar and replace the orange zest with ½ teaspoon grated fresh ginger. Omit the almond extract.

Serving size: 1 cookie Calories: 51; Protein: <1g; Total fat: 0; Saturated fat: 0g; Carbohydrates: 13g; Fiber: 0g; Sodium: 17mg

HEAL

REINTRODUCE

Peanut Butter Cookies

PREP TIME: 10 MINUTES; COOK TIME: 10 MINUTES

If you're longing for a more traditional cookie, try this recipe. It is so easy, and it yields tasty peanut butter cookies. The best part is it has only three ingredients, so the cookies are super quick to put together, and in less than 10 minutes you can have warm cookies. Due to the fat content and calories, these cookies should just be an occasional treat.

MAKES 6

5-INGREDIENT
30-MINUTE

1 cup peanut butter
1 cup brown sugar
1 large egg

1. Preheat the oven to 350°F. Line a baking sheet with parchment paper or grease the baking sheet.

2. In a medium bowl, cream together all the ingredients until well mixed.

3. Spoon the batter into 6 portions on the prepared baking sheet.

4. Bake until the bottoms begin to brown, 6 to 8 minutes.

FLAVOR BOOST: Sprinkle each cookie with 1 teaspoon chopped peanuts for a bit of crunch.

Serving size: 1 cookie Calories: 355; Protein: 12g; Total fat: 22g; Saturated fat: 5g; Carbohydrates: 32g; Fiber: 3g; Sodium: 24mg

Banana Pudding

PREP TIME: 5 MINUTES (PLUS CHILLING TIME); COOK TIME: 10 MINUTES

Banana pudding is really a misnomer here—this dessert is actually vanilla pudding with bananas on the bottom. You can either use fresh bananas or, for added flavor, use Brûléed Bananas (page 186). This is a creamy, sweet treat you're sure to love. SERVES 4

5-INGREDIENT

¼ cup sugar

2 tablespoons cornstarch

1 cup lactose-free nonfat milk

½ teaspoon vanilla extract

1 banana, peeled and sliced

1. In a small bowl, whisk together the sugar and cornstarch.

2. In a small saucepan, bring the milk to a simmer over medium heat, stirring.

3. Pour the sugar mixture slowly into the hot milk, whisking constantly.

4. Cook, stirring constantly, until the mixture coats the back of a spoon, 3 to 5 minutes.

5. Remove from the heat and whisk in the vanilla.

6. Divide the banana slices among four ramekins.

7. Top with the pudding and refrigerate until ready to serve.

FLAVOR BOOST: Substitute ½ teaspoon rum extract for the vanilla and add ¼ teaspoon ground cinnamon to the sugar and cornstarch mixture.

SUBSTITUTION: For REINTRODUCE, replace the banana with another fruit, such as ¼ cup chopped apple, ½ cup sliced strawberries, or ¼ cup blueberries.

Serving size: ¼ cup Calories: 112; Protein: 3g; Total fat: <1; Saturated fat: 0g; Carbohydrates: 26g; Fiber: <1g; Sodium: 33mg

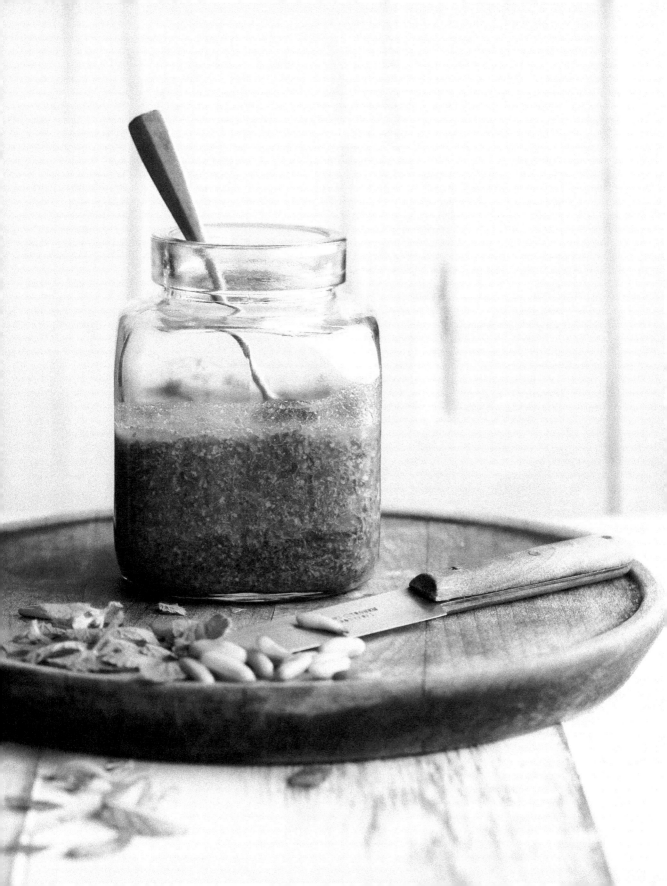

10

Sauces and Condiments

Beef Broth 194

Poultry Broth 195

Papaya Vinaigrette 196

Tartar Sauce 197

Burger Sauce 198

Lemon Yogurt Sauce 199

Creamy Herbed Dressing 200

Walnut-Basil Pesto 201

Kale, Oregano, and
   Pine Nut Pesto 202

Basil Dressing 203

Stir-Fry Sauce 204

Oregano and Parsley
   Chimichurri 205

Cantaloupe Salsa 206

Guacamole 207

Yogurt Sour Cream 208

Garlic Oil 209

Kale, Oregano, and Pine Nut Pesto, page 202

Beef Broth

PREP TIME: 10 MINUTES; COOK TIME: 12 HOURS (SLOW COOKER)

Using your slow cooker yields a rich, flavorful beef broth. The longer you simmer it, the more flavorful it is, but don't simmer for more than about 24 hours because after that period it can grow bitter. YIELD: ABOUT 8 CUPS

5-INGREDIENT

3 pounds beef bones

3 carrots,
  roughly chopped

1 fennel bulb,
  roughly chopped

1 bay leaf

1 rosemary sprig

1 thyme sprig

9 cups water

1. In a slow cooker, combine all the ingredients
2. Cover and simmer on low for 12 to 24 hours.
3. Strain out the solids. Refrigerate overnight.
4. In the morning, skim and discard the fat. Store in one-cup servings in the freezer for up to six months.

COOKING TIP: You can also simmer this on the stove top. Cover and simmer for three hours in a large pot.

Serving size: 1 cup Calories: 20; Protein: 2g; Total fat: 0g; Saturated fat: 0g; Carbohydrates: 2g; Fiber: 0g; Sodium: 140mg

Poultry Broth

PREP TIME: 10 MINUTES; COOK TIME: 4 HOURS

You can use chicken or turkey bones in this broth. For example, if you eat a rotisserie chicken, save the bones in the freezer to use in your broth. If desired, you can use low-meat cuts, such as backs, necks, or wings. You can also make it in the slow cooker (just go for 12 hours on low instead of 4). Store the broth in one-cup servings in your freezer for up to a year, and you can just thaw what you need as you need it. SERVES 8

5-INGREDIENT

ONE-PAN

1 carrot, peeled
   and chopped

1 leek, green part only,
   roughly chopped and
   washed (see headnote,
   page 110)

1 celery stalk,
   roughly chopped

2 pounds poultry bones

9 cups water

1. In a large pot, combine all the ingredients.

2. Bring to a simmer over medium-high heat, then lower the heat to low and simmer for 4 hours.

3. Strain the vegetables and bones from the broth and store the broth in the refrigerator overnight.

4. Skim the fat that has solidified on top of the broth and discard it. Store the broth in 1-cup servings in the freezer until you're ready to use it.

FLAVOR BOOST: You can also use this with beef bones to make a beef broth. For a more aromatic broth, add a sprig of thyme to the broth as you simmer it.

SUBSTITUTION: For REINTRODUCE, replace the leek with ½ small onion, roughly chopped.

Serving size: 1 cup Calories: 10; Protein: 0g; Total fat: 0g; Saturated fat: 0g; Carbohydrates: 3g; Fiber: 0g; Sodium: 40mg

Papaya Vinaigrette

PREP TIME: 10 MINUTES

This papaya vinaigrette is a great salad dressing, and it's also a delicious meat marinade if you add 2 tablespoons coconut aminos and ¼ teaspoon fish sauce to it. It will keep for up to 3 days in the refrigerator, so you'll most likely want to make small batches. SERVES 4

5-INGREDIENT
30-MINUTE
ONE-PAN

½ papaya, chopped

1 tablespoon olive oil

½ teaspoon grated
  lemon zest

1 tablespoon chopped
  fresh thyme

½ teaspoon sea salt

¼ cup water (optional)

In a blender or food processor, combine the papaya, olive oil, lemon zest, thyme, and salt. Process until smooth, thinning with the water, as needed.

FLAVOR BOOST: Add ½ teaspoon ground mustard.

Serving size: 2 tablespoons Calories: 47; Protein: <1g; Total fat: 4g; Saturated fat: <1g; Carbohydrates: 4g; Fiber: 1g; Sodium: 235mg

Tartar Sauce

PREP TIME: 5 MINUTES

Regular tartar sauce can be a bit high in acid and fat, but this version serves as a workable substitute. It's very easy to make and can add good flavor to fish or burgers. It will keep in the refrigerator for up to 5 days. SERVES 4

5-INGREDIENT
30-MINUTE
ONE-PAN

½ cup lactose-free nonfat plain yogurt

2 tablespoons chopped fresh dill

1 teaspoon grated lemon zest

½ teaspoon sea salt

In a small bowl, mix all the ingredients until well combined.

SUBSTITUTION: To make this suitable for the STOP plan, replace the yogurt with ½ cup tofu and 2 tablespoons lactose-free nonfat milk. Blend in a food processor or blender.

Serving size: 2 tablespoons Calories: 20; Protein: 2g; Total fat: <1g; Saturated fat: <1g; Carbohydrates: 3g; Fiber: <1g; Sodium: 259mg

HEAL

REINTRODUCE

Burger Sauce

PREP TIME: 5 MINUTES

This savory sauce is great on burgers, and it also makes a delicious dip for Baked Potato Chips (page 176) or Sweet Potato French Fries (page 96). It will keep in the refrigerator for up to 5 days. Coconut aminos is a stand-in for soy sauce. If you can't find it in the grocery store or health food store, it is available from online retailers. SERVES 4

5-INGREDIENT
30-MINUTE
ONE-PAN

½ cup lactose-free nonfat
   plain yogurt

1 tablespoon
   coconut aminos

½ teaspoon fish sauce

2 tablespoons
   brown sugar

2 tablespoons chopped
   fresh thyme

In a small bowl, mix all the ingredients until well combined.

SUBSTITUTION: For a sauce with Asian flair, replace the thyme with chopped fresh cilantro and add ½ teaspoon grated lime zest and 1 teaspoon grated fresh ginger. For REINTRODUCE, add 1 tablespoon chopped fresh chives and ¼ garlic clove, finely chopped.

Serving size: 2 tablespoons Calories: 39; Protein: 2g; Total fat: <1g; Saturated fat: <1g; Carbohydrates: 8g; Fiber: <1g; Sodium: 134mg

Lemon Yogurt Sauce

PREP TIME: 5 MINUTES

To add a fresh, deliciously lemony flavor to fish or burgers, this sauce is perfect. It will store in the refrigerator for up to 5 days. SERVES 4

5-INGREDIENT

30-MINUTE

ONE-PAN

½ cup lactose-free nonfat
plain yogurt

1 teaspoon grated
lemon zest

¼ teaspoon sea salt

In a small bowl, mix all the ingredients until well combined.

SUBSTITUTION: To make this suitable for STOP, replace the yogurt with ½ cup tofu and 2 tablespoons lactose-free nonfat milk. Blend in a food processor or blender until smooth.

Serving size: 2 tablespoons Calories: 17; Protein: 2g;
Total fat: <1g; Saturated fat: <1g; Carbohydrates: 3g; Fiber: 0g;
Sodium: 138mg

Creamy Herbed Dressing

PREP TIME: 5 MINUTES

If you're a ranch dressing fan, this is a tasty substitute. It's made with a variety of herbs to give it a fresh flavor. You can thin it with a little lactose-free nonfat milk to achieve the desired thickness, if desired. SERVES 4

5-INGREDIENT

30-MINUTE

ONE-PAN

½ cup lactose-free nonfat plain yogurt

1 teaspoon grated lemon zest

1 tablespoon chopped fresh parsley

1 tablespoon chopped fresh thyme

1 teaspoon chopped fresh rosemary

¼ teaspoon sea salt

In a small bowl, mix all the ingredients until well combined.

SUBSTITUTION: To make this suitable for STOP, replace the yogurt with ½ cup silken tofu and 2 tablespoons milk and blend in a food processor or blender until smooth. Adjust the consistency with additional milk. For REINTRODUCE, add 1 tablespoon chopped fresh chives and ½ garlic clove, finely minced.

Serving size: 2 tablespoons Calories: 17; Protein: 2g; Total fat: <1g; Saturated fat: <1g; Carbohydrates: 3g; Fiber: <1g; Sodium: 139mg

Walnut-Basil Pesto

PREP TIME: 5 MINUTES

This quick pesto is delicious on gluten-free pasta. It's equally tasty as a sandwich spread, on burgers, or on a plain protein such as a piece of fish or chicken. It's a great way to add instant flavor to any food. SERVES 2

5-INGREDIENT
30-MINUTE
ONE-PAN

½ cup fresh basil leaves

¼ cup grated
  Parmesan cheese

¼ cup walnuts

2 tablespoons olive oil

1 teaspoon grated
  lemon zest

In a blender or food processor, combine all the ingredients and pulse 20 times, or until chopped and combined.

SUBSTITUTION: If you're not a fan of walnuts, replace them with pine nuts for a more classic pesto. For REINTRODUCE, add ½ garlic clove, minced.

Serving size: ¼ cup Calories: 189; Protein: 5g; Total fat: 19g; Saturated fat: 4g; Carbohydrates: 1g; Fiber: 1g; Sodium: 132mg

STOP

HEAL

REINTRODUCE

Kale, Oregano, and Pine Nut Pesto

PREP TIME: 5 MINUTES

Whether you use this on fish, chicken, gluten-free pasta, or even eggs, this bright green pesto adds bold flavor and brings the nutrition of kale. SERVES 2

5-INGREDIENT
30-MINUTE
ONE-PAN

1 cup roughly
   chopped kale

¼ cup fresh
   oregano leaves

¼ cup pine nuts

2 tablespoons olive oil

1 teaspoon grated
   orange zest

In a blender or food processor, combine all the ingredients and pulse 20 times, or until chopped and combined.

SUBSTITUTION: For REINTRODUCE, add ½ garlic clove, minced.

Serving size: ¼ cup Calories: 171; Protein: 2g; Total fat: 16g; Saturated fat: 3g; Carbohydrates: 7g; Fiber: 1g; Sodium: 15mg

Basil Dressing

PREP TIME: 5 MINUTES

Orange is a perfect complement to the freshness of the basil in this dressing. Enjoy it on a salad, or serve it as a topper for protein or veggies. It will keep for up to 3 days in the refrigerator. SERVES 4

30-MINUTE
ONE-PAN

¼ cup lactose-free plain nonfat yogurt

2 tablespoons lactose-free nonfat milk

1 tablespoon olive oil

2 tablespoons chopped fresh basil

½ teaspoon grated orange zest

½ teaspoon salt

In a small bowl, mix all the ingredients until well combined.

SUBSTITUTION: To make this suitable for STOP, replace the yogurt with ¼ cup tofu and 2 tablespoons nonfat milk. Blend in a food processor or blender until smooth. Adjust the consistency with additional milk.

Serving size: 2 tablespoons Calories: 44; Protein: 1g; Total fat: 4g; Saturated fat: <1g; Carbohydrates: 2g; Fiber: 0g; Sodium: 306mg

Stir-Fry Sauce

PREP TIME: 5 MINUTES

Add this sauce to any stir-fry for additional flavor. It uses coconut aminos in place of soy sauce. If you can't find coconut aminos at your local grocery store or health food store (it's in the soy sauce aisle), you can get it from online retailers. SERVES 4

5-INGREDIENT
30-MINUTE
ONE-PAN

**2 tablespoons
  coconut aminos**

**¼ cup Simple Vegetable
  Broth (page 108)**

**½ teaspoon fish sauce
  (omit if vegetarian)**

1 teaspoon cornstarch

1 teaspoon ground ginger

In a small bowl, whisk all the ingredients together to combine.

FLAVOR BOOST: Add 1 tablespoon pure maple syrup for a hint of sweetness.

SUBSTITUTION: For REINTRODUCE, add ½ garlic clove, finely minced.

Serving size: 2 tablespoons Calories: 12; Protein: <1g; Total fat: 0g; Saturated fat: 0g; Carbohydrates: 3g; Fiber: <1g; Sodium: 163mg

Oregano and Parsley Chimichurri

PREP TIME: 5 MINUTES

This chopped herb condiment is delicious on meat, poultry, and fish. It is also flavorful as a sandwich or burger spread. It doesn't store well, so make small batches for best results. SERVES 2

5-INGREDIENT
30-MINUTE
ONE-PAN

¼ cup chopped
   fresh oregano

¼ cup chopped
   fresh parsley

2 tablespoons olive oil

1 teaspoon grated
   lemon zest

½ teaspoon sea salt

In a blender or food processor, combine all the ingredients and pulse 20 times, or until the herbs are well chopped.

SUBSTITUTION: To give this a Southwestern flair, replace the oregano with ¼ cup chopped fresh cilantro and replace the lemon zest with lime zest. Add a pinch of ground cumin. For REINTRODUCE, add ½ garlic clove, finely minced.

Serving size: ¼ cup Calories: 133; Protein: 1g; Total fat: 14g; Saturated fat: 2g; Carbohydrates: 3g; Fiber: 1g; Sodium: 474mg

Cantaloupe Salsa

PREP TIME: 5 MINUTES

This salsa is incredibly simple; it has only five ingredients, but it adds wonderful bright-ness and freshness to foods. Top fish with it, put it on a burger, or serve it with chips as a dip. It will keep in the refrigerator for about 2 days. SERVES 2

5-INGREDIENT
30-MINUTE
ONE-PAN

½ **cup chopped fresh
cantaloupe**

¼ **cup chopped fresh
cilantro**

1 **teaspoon grated
lime zest**

½ **teaspoon ground cumin**

½ **teaspoon sea salt**

In a small bowl, mix all the ingredients until well combined.

SUBSTITUTION: For REINTRODUCE, replace the cantaloupe with ½ cup chopped mango and add ¼ red onion, minced.

Serving size: ¼ cup Calories: 16; Protein: <1g; Total fat: <1g; Saturated fat: 0g; Carbohydrates: 4g; Fiber: <1g; Sodium: 476mg

Guacamole

PREP TIME: 5 MINUTES

On all three plans, you can safely have about ⅛ avocado. Therefore, it's important you limit your serving sizes of this guacamole, unless you're on the STOP plan, in which case you can have a bit more. This recipe doesn't keep well. If you do store it, lay plastic wrap directly on the surface of the guacamole to keep the avocado from oxidizing. SERVES 4

5-INGREDIENT
30-MINUTE
ONE-PAN

½ ripe avocado, peeled and pitted

2 tablespoons chopped fresh cilantro

½ teaspoon grated lime zest

½ teaspoon ground cumin

½ teaspoon sea salt

In a small bowl, combine all the ingredients and mash with a fork.

FLAVOR BOOST: Add ½ teaspoon ground coriander.

SUBSTITUTION: For REINTRODUCE, add 2 tablespoons minced red onion.

Serving size: 2 tablespoons Calories: 52; Protein: <1g; Total fat: 5g; Saturated fat: 1g; Carbohydrates: 2g; Fiber: 2g; Sodium: 236mg

STOP

HEAL

REINTRODUCE

Yogurt Sour Cream

PREP TIME: 5 MINUTES

Sour cream tends to be pretty high in fat, and it contains lactose, so for this version we use lactose-free nonfat plain yogurt and add spices for a Southwestern flair. Try it on tacos or a baked potato. SERVES 4

5-INGREDIENT
30-MINUTE
ONE-PAN

½ cup lactose-free nonfat
plain yogurt

½ teaspoon grated
lime zest

½ teaspoon ground
coriander

½ teaspoon ground cumin

½ teaspoon sea salt

In a small bowl, mix all the ingredients until well combined.

SUBSTITUTION: To make this suitable for STOP, replace the yogurt with ½ cup tofu and 2 tablespoons nonfat milk. Blend in a food processor or blender until smooth, adjusting the consistency with additional milk if needed.

Serving size: 2 tablespoons Calories: 23; Protein: 2g;
Total fat: <1g; Saturated fat: <1g; Carbohydrates: 2g; Fiber: <1g;
Sodium: 256mg

Garlic Oil

PREP TIME: 5 MINUTES COOK TIME: 10 MINUTES

This garlic oil is a good add-in for recipes if you find garlic doesn't cause your acid reflux to flare but you are sensitive to FODMAPs and need to avoid them. Make it in small batches, since it will keep for only about three days. Allow it to cool completely, and you can whisk it into vinaigrettes or use as a cooking oil in recipes—it will impart garlic flavor without the FODMAPs. SERVES 4

¼ cup extra-virgin olive oil

3 garlic cloves, sliced

In a small saucepan on the lowest heat setting, simmer the garlic in the olive oil for 10 minutes. Allow to cool completely and strain out the garlic.

FLAVOR BOOST: The trick here is to simmer the oil without boiling it. To do this, you need to set your stove on as low a setting as possible. You may also need to lift the pan away from the stove by making a ring of wadded aluminum foil and placing it on the burner with the pan on the foil.

Serving size: 1 tablespoon Calories: 108; Protein: 0g; Total fat: 13g; Saturated Fat: 2g; Carbohydrates: 0g; Fiber: 0g; Sodium: 0mg

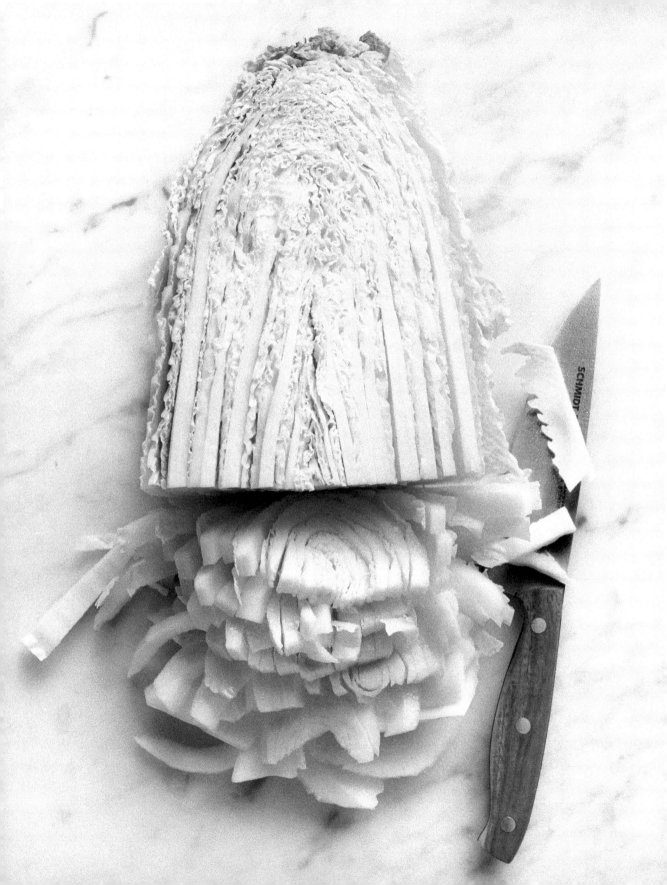

The FDA's pH Food Lists

VEGETABLES

FOOD	pH
Artichokes, fresh	5.6
Artichokes, canned	5.7 to 6.0
Asparagus, fresh	6.1 to 6.7
Asparagus, canned	5.2 to 5.3
Beans, green	4.6
Beans, lima	6.5
Beets, fresh	4.9 to 5.6
Beets, canned	4.9
Brussels sprouts	6.0 to 6.3
Cabbage, green	5.4 to 6.9
Cabbage, red	5.4 to 6.0
Cabbage, savoy	6.3
Cabbage, white	6.2
Carrots, fresh	4.9 to 5.2
Carrots, canned	5.2
Cauliflower	5.6
Celery	5.7 to 6.0
Corn, fresh	6.0 to 7.5
Corn, canned	6.0
Cucumbers	5.1 to 5.7
Cucumbers, pickled	3.2 to 3.5
Eggplant	4.5 to 5.3
Hominy	6.0
Kale	6.4 to 6.8

VEGETABLES

FOOD	pH
Kohlrabi	5.7 to 5.8
Leeks	5.5 to 6.0
Lettuce	5.8 to 6.0
Mushrooms	6.2
Okra	5.5 to 6.4
Olives, black	6.0 to 6.5
Olives, green	3.6 to 3.8
Onions, red	5.3 to 5.8
Onions, white	5.4 to 5.8
Onions, yellow	5.4 to 5.6
Parsnips	5.3
Peas, fresh	5.8 to 7.0
Peas, frozen	6.4 to 6.7
Peas, canned	5.7 to 6.0
Peppers, bell	5.2
Potatoes, russet	6.1
Potatoes, sweet	5.3 to 5.6
Pumpkin	4.8 to 5.2
Radishes, red	5.8 to 6.5
Radishes, white	5.5 to 5.7
Rhubarb	3.1 to 3.4
Sauerkraut	3.5 to 3.6
Spinach, fresh	5.5 to 6.8
Spinach, frozen	6.3 to 6.5

VEGETABLES

FOOD	pH
Squash	5.5 to 6.0
Tomatoes, fresh	4.2 to 4.9
Tomatoes, canned	3.5 to 4.7
Tomato juice	4.1 to 4.2
Tomato paste	3.5 to 4.7
Turnips	5.2 to 5.5
Zucchini	5.8 to 6.1

HERBS

FOOD	pH
Chives	5.2 to 6.1
Horseradish	5.3
Parsley	5.7 to 6.0
Sorrel	3.7

GRAINS & LEGUMES

FOOD	pH
Beans, kidney	5.4 to 6.0
Bread	5.3 to 5.8
Cake	5.2 to 8.0
Crackers	7.0 to 8.5
Flour	6.0 to 6.3
Lentils	6.3 to 6.8
Rice, brown	6.2 to 6.7
Rice, white	6.0 to 6.7
Rice, wild	6.0 to 6.4

FRUITS

FOOD	pH
Apples	3.3 to 3.9
Apple juice	3.4 to 4.0
Applesauce	3.3 to 3.6
Apricots, fresh	3.3 to 4.0
Apricots, dried	3.6 to 4.0
Apricots, canned	3.7
Bananas	4.5 to 5.2
Blackberries	3.2 to 4.5
Blueberries, fresh	3.7
Blueberries, frozen	3.1 to 3.4
Cantaloupe	6.2 to 7.1
Cherries	3.2 to 4.1
Cranberry sauce	2.4
Cranberry juice	2.3 to 2.5
Dates	6.3 to 6.6
Figs	4.6
Grapefruit	3.0 to 3.3
Grapes	3.4 to 4.5
Lemons	2.2 to 2.4
Limes	1.8 to 2.0
Mango	3.9 to 4.6
Melons, honeydew	6.3 to 6.7
Nectarines	3.9
Oranges	3.1 to 4.1
Orange juice	3.6 to 4.3

FRUITS

FOOD	pH
Papaya	5.2 to 5.7
Peaches, fresh	3.4 to 3.6
Peaches, jarred	4.2
Peaches, canned	4.9
Persimmons	5.4 to 5.8
Pineapple, fresh	3.3 to 5.2
Pineapple, canned	3.5
Plums	2.8 to 4.6
Pomegranates	3.0
Prunes	3.1 to 5.4
Prune juice	3.7
Raspberries	3.2 to 3.7
Strawberries, fresh	3.0 to 3.5
Strawberries, frozen	2.3 to 3.0
Tangerines	4.0
Watermelon	5.2 to 5.8

DAIRY

FOOD	pH
Butter	6.1 to 6.4
Buttermilk	4.5
Milk	6.3 to 8.5
Cream	6.5
Cheese, Camembert	7.4
Cheese, Cheddar	5.9
Cheese, cottage	5.0

DAIRY

FOOD	pH
Cheese, cream	4.9
Cheese, Edam	5.4
Cheese, Roquefort	5.5 to 5.9
Cheese, Swiss	5.1 to 6.6
Eggs, whites	7.0 to 9.0
Eggs, yolks	6.4
Eggs, whole	7.1 to 7.9

MEAT, POULTRY, FISH

FOOD	pH
Beef, ground	5.1 to 6.2
Beef, steak	5.8 to 7.0
Chicken	6.5 to 6.7
Clams	6.5
Crab	7.0
Fish	6.6 to 7.3
Ham	5.9 to 6.1
Lamb	5.4 to 6.7
Oysters	4.8 to 6.3
Pork	5.3 to 6.9
Salmon	6.1 to 6.3
Shrimp	6.8 to 7.0
Tuna	5.2 to 6.1
Turkey	5.7 to 6.8
Veal	6.0
Whitefish	5.5

OTHER

FOOD	pH
Cider	2.9 to 3.3
Cocoa	6.3
Corn syrup	5.0
Cornstarch	4.0 to 7.0
Ginger ale	2.0 to 4.0
Honey	3.9
Jam	3.1 to 3.5
Mayonnaise	4.2 to 4.5
Molasses	5.0 to 5.5
Raisins	3.8 to 4.0
Sugar	5.0 to 6.0
Vinegar	2.0 to 3.5
Yeast	3.0 to 3.5

The Dirty Dozen
and the Clean Fifteen™

A nonprofit environmental watchdog organization called Environmental Working Group (EWG) looks at data supplied by the U.S. Department of Agriculture (USDA) and the Food and Drug Administration (FDA) about pesticide residues. Each year it compiles a list of the best and worst pesticide loads found in commercial crops. You can use these lists to decide which fruits and vegetables to buy organic to minimize your exposure to pesticides and which produce is considered safe enough to buy conventionally. This does not mean they are pesticide-free, though, so wash these fruits and vegetables thoroughly.

These lists change every year, so make sure you look up the most recent one before you fill your shopping cart. You'll find the most recent lists as well as a guide to pesticides in produce at EWG.org/FoodNews.

DIRTY DOZEN

Apples

Celery

Cherry tomatoes

Cucumbers

Grapes

Nectarines (imported)

Peaches

Potatoes

Snap peas (imported)

Spinach

Strawberries

Sweet bell peppers

In addition to the Dirty Dozen, the EWG added two types of produce contaminated with highly toxic organophosphate insecticides:

Kale/collard greens

Hot peppers

CLEAN FIFTEEN

Asparagus

Avocados

Cabbage

Cantaloupes (domestic)

Cauliflower

Eggplants

Grapefruits

Kiwis

Mangoes

Onions

Papayas

Pineapples

Sweet corn

Sweet peas (frozen)

Sweet potatoes

Measurements and Conversions

VOLUME EQUIVALENTS (LIQUID)

US STANDARD	US STANDARD (OUNCES)	METRIC (APPROX)
2 tablespoons	1 fl. oz.	30 mL
¼ cup	2 fl. oz.	60 mL
½ cup	4 fl. oz.	120 mL
1 cup	8 fl. oz.	240 mL
1½ cups	12 fl. oz	355 mL
2 cups or 1 pint	16 fl. oz.	475 mL
4 cups or 1 quart	32 fl. oz.	1 L
1 gallon	128 fl. oz.	4 L

OVEN TEMPERATURES

FAHRENHEIT (F)	CELSIUS (C) (APPROX)
250°F	120°C
300°F	150°C
325°F	165°C
350°F	180°C
375°F	190°C
400°F	200°C
425°F	220°C
450°F	230°C

VOLUME EQUIVALENTS (DRY)

US STANDARD	METRIC (APPROX)
⅛ teaspoon	0.5 mL
¼ teaspoon	1 mL
½ teaspoon	2 mL
¾ teaspoon	4 mL
1 teaspoon	5 mL
1 tablespoon	15 mL
¼ cup	59 mL
⅓ cup	79 mL
½ cup	118 mL
⅔ cup	156 mL
¾ cup	177 mL
1 cup	235 mL
2 cups or 1 pint	475 mL
3 cups	700 mL
4 cups or 1 quart	1 L

WEIGHT EQUIVALENTS

US STANDARD	METRIC (APPROX)
½ ounce	15 g
1 ounce	30 g
2 ounces	60 g
4 ounces	115 g
8 ounces	225 g
12 ounces	340 g
16 ounces or 1 pound	455 g

References

Austin, Gregory L., Michelle T. Thiny, Eric C. Westman, William S. Yancy, and Nicholas J. Shaheen. "A Very Low-Carbohydrate Diet Improves Gastroesophageal Reflux and Its Symptoms." *Digestive Diseases and Sciences* 51, no. 8 (2006): 1307–312. doi:10.1007/s10620-005-9027-7.

Banoo, H. and N. Nusrat. "Implications of Low Stomach Acid: An Update" *Rama University Journal of Medical Sciences* 2, no. 2 (2016): 16–26.

CNN. "The Most-Prescribed Medications." Accessed January 1, 2018. http://www.cnn.com/2016/11/25/health/gallery/most-prescribed-medications/index.html.

Dr. Oz Show. "Silent Reflux: A Hidden Epidemic." Accessed January 1, 2018. http://www.doctoroz.com/article/silent-reflux-epidemic.

Drugs.com. "U.S. Pharmaceutical Sales: Q4 2013." Accessed January 1, 2018. https://www.drugs.com/stats/top100/sales.

El-Omar, E. M., K. Oien, A. El-Nujumi, D. Gillen, A. Wirz, S. Dahill, C. Williams, J. E. Ardill, and K. E. McColl. "*Helicobacter Pylori* Infection and Chronic Gastric Acid Hyposecretion." *Gastroenterology* 113, no. 1 (1997): 15–24. doi:10.1016/s0016-5085(97)70075-1.

Fu, Jingyuan, Marc Jan Bonder, María Carmen Cenit, Ettje F. Tigchelaar, Astrid Maatman, Jackie AM Dekens, Eelke Brandsma et al. "The gut microbiome contributes to a substantial proportion of the variation in blood lipids." Circulation Research 117, no. 9 (2015): 817-824.

Greenwald, David A. "Aging, the Gastrointestinal Tract, and Risk of Acid-Related Disease." *American Journal of Medicine Supplements* 117, no. 5 (2004): 8–13. doi:10.1016/j.amjmed.2004.07.019.

Kelly, Gregory. "Hydrochloric Acid: Physiological Functions and Clinical Implications" *Alternative Medicine Review*, 2, no. 2 (1997): 116–127.

Khalifa, Mohammed, Radwa Sharaf, and Ramy Aziz. "*Helicobacter Pylori*: A Poor Man's Gut Pathogen?" *Gut Pathogens* 2, no. 1 (2010): 2. doi:10.1186/1757-4749-2-2.

Koufman, Jamie, Jordan Stern, and Marc Bauer. *Dropping Acid: The Reflux Diet Cookbook and Cure*. Reflux Cookbooks, 2015.

Krasinski, Stephen D., Robert M. Russell, I. Michael Samloff, Robert A. Jacob, Gerard E. Dallal, Robert B. McGandy, and Stuart C. Hartz. "Fundic Atrophic Gastritis in an Elderly Population: Effect on Hemoglobin and Several Serum Nutritional Indicators." *Journal of the American Geriatrics Society* 34, no. 11 (1986): 800–06. doi:10.1111/j.1532-5415.1986.tb03985.x.

Kresser, Chris. "More Evidence to Support the Theory That GERD Is Caused by Bacterial Overgrowth." Accessed January 10, 2018. https://chriskresser.com/more-evidence-to-support-the-theory-that-gerd-is-caused-by-bacterial-overgrowth/.

Kresser, Chris. "The Hidden Causes of Heartburn and GERD." Accessed January 10, 2018. https://chriskresser.com/the-hidden-causes-of-heartburn-and-gerd/.

Kresser, Chris. "What Everybody Ought to Know (But Doesn't) about Heartburn and GERD." Accessed January 10, 2018. https://chriskresser.com/what-everybody-ought-to-know-but-doesnt-about-heartburn-gerd/.

Monash University. "FODMAPs and Irritable Bowel Syndrome." Accessed February 4, 2018. https://www.monashfodmap.com/about-fodmap-and-ibs/.

National Institute of Diabetes and Digestive and Kidney Diseases. "Digestive Diseases Statistics for the United States." Accessed January 1, 2018. https://www.niddk.nih.gov/health-information/health-statistics/digestive-diseases#specific.

Nutrition Reviews "Gastric Balance: Heartburn Not Always Caused by Excess Acid." Accessed January 28, 2018. https://nutritionreview.org/2013/04/gastric-balance-heartburn-caused-excess-acid/.

Panahi, Yunes, Hossein Khedmat, Ghasem Valizadegan, Reza Mohtashami, and Amirhossein Sahebkar. "Efficacy and Safety of Aloe Vera Syrup for the Treatment of Gastroesophageal Reflux Disease: A Pilot Randomized Positive-Controlled Trial." *Journal of Traditional Chinese Medicine* 35, no. 6 (2015): 632-36. doi:10.1016/s0254-6272(15)30151–5.

Robillard, Norman. *Fast Tract Digestion: Heartburn*. Watertown, MA: Self Health Publishing, 2012.

Sharp, George S., and H. William Fister. "The Diagnosis and Treatment of Achlorhydria: Ten-Year Study." *Journal of the American Geriatrics Society* 15, no. 8 (1967): 786–91. doi:10.1111/j.1532-5415.1967.tb02312.x.

Sugerman, Harvey J. "Increased Intra-abdominal Pressure and GERD/Barrett's Esophagus." *Gastroenterology* 133, no. 6 (2007): 2075. doi:10.1053/j.gastro.2007.10.017.

Theisen, Jörg, Dhiren Nehra, Diane Dhiren, Jan Johansson, Jeffrey Hagen, Peter Crookes, Steven DeMeester, Cedric Bremner, Tom DeMeester, and Jeffrey Peters. "Suppression of Gastric Acid Secretion in Patients with Gastroesophageal Reflux Disease Results in Gastric Bacterial Overgrowth and Deconjugation of Bile Acids." *Journal of Gastrointestinal Surgery* 4, no. 1 (2000): 50–54. doi:10.1016/s1091-255x(00)80032-3.

World Gastroenterology Organization. "WGO Handbook on Heartburn: A Global Perspective." World Digestive Health Day, May 29, 2015. Accessed January 1, 2018. http://www.worldgastroenterology.org/UserFiles/file/WDHD-2015-handbook-final.pdf.

Wormsley, K. G., and M. Grossman. "Maximal Histalog Test in Control Subjects and Patients with Peptic Ulcer." *Gut* 6, no. 5 (1965): 427–435.

Yarandi, Shadi Sadeghi, S. Nasseri-Moghaddam, P. Mostajabi, and R. Malekzadeh. "Overlapping Gastroesophageal Reflux Disease and Irritable Bowel Syndrome: Increased Dysfunctional Symptoms." *World Journal of Gastroenterology* 16, no. 10 (2010): 1232–238.

Resources

BOOKS

Catsos, Patsy. *The IBS Elimination Diet and Cookbook: The Proven Low-FODMAP Plan for Eating Well and Feeling Great.* Harmony Books, 2017.

Frazier, Karen. *The Easy Acid Reflux Cookbook: Comforting 30-Minute Recipes to Soothe GERD and LPR.* Berkeley, CA: Rockridge Press, 2017.

Koufman, Jamie, Jordan Stern, and Marc Bauer. *Dropping Acid: The Reflux Diet Cookbook and Cure.* Place of publication not identified: Reflux Cookbooks, 2015.

Robillard, Norman. *Fast Tract Digestion: Heartburn.* Watertown, MA: Self Health Publishing, 2012.

Wright, Jonathan V., and Lane Lenard. *Why Stomach Acid Is Good for You: Natural Relief from Heartburn, Indigestion, Reflux, and GERD.* New York: M. Evans, 2001.

WEBSITES

American College of Gastroenterology. "Acid Reflux." http://patients.gi.org/topics/acid-reflux/

Monash University. "FODMAPs and Irritable Bowel Syndrome." https://www.monashfodmap.com/about-fodmap-and-ibs/

National Institute of Diabetes and Digestive and Kidney Diseases. "Acid Reflux (GER and GERD) in Adults." https://www.niddk.nih.gov/health-information/digestive-diseases/acid-reflux-ger-gerd-adults

APPS

Acid Reflux Diet Helper by Duncan Donaldson. https://itunes.apple.com/us
/app/acid-reflux-diet-helper/id1230575459?mt=8

Fast Tract Diet App by Norm Robillard. https://itunes.apple.com/us/app
/fast-tract-diet/id1062915865?mt=8

Monash University FODMAP Diet App by Monash University. https://itunes
.apple.com/au/app/monash-university-low-fodmap-diet/id586149216?mt=8

Recipe Index

A

Almond Meringue Cookies, 189
Apple Compote Smoothie, 75
Artichoke Purée, 97
Asian Veggie and
    Tofu Stir-Fry, 120

B

Baked Avocado and Egg, 85
Baked Chicken Tenders, 144
Baked Potato Chips, 176
Banana and Melon Salad, 188
Banana-Flax Smoothie, 70
Banana Ice Cream, 187
Banana Pancakes, 80
Banana Pudding, 191
Basil Dressing, 203
Beef Broth, 194
Beef Tacos, 161
Breaded Crispy Shrimp, 134
Broccoli and Cheese
    Baked Potato, 115
Brown Rice and Peanut
    Lettuce Wraps, 122
Brown Rice and
    Tofu with Kale, 125
Brûléed Bananas, 186
Burger Sauce, 198
Butternut Risotto, 124

C

Cantaloupe Salsa, 206
Carrots with Herbed
    Yogurt Dip, 177
Chia Breakfast Pudding
    with Cantaloupe, 73
Chicken Noodle Soup, 143
Chopped Kale Salad, 104
Cinnamon-Sugar Popcorn, 174

Cooling Cucumber Soup, 109
Corn Porridge with
    Maple and Raisins, 77
Crab Cakes with
    Tartar Sauce, 132
Creamed Spinach, 100
Cream of Broccoli Soup, 113
Creamy Herbed Dressing, 200
Creamy Pumpkin Soup, 112
Cucumber Rounds with
    Shrimp Salad, 175

D

Deviled Eggs, 172

E

Easy Tuna Melt, 138
Easy Turkey Burgers, 148

F

Fisherman's Stew, 142
Fish Tacos with
    Guacamole, 141
Flank Steak with
    Chimichurri, 162
French Toast, 79
Fried Egg Sandwich, 129
Fruit and Yogurt Parfait, 74

G

Garlic Oil, 209
Grated Carrot and
    Raisin Salad, 179
Green Aloe Vera Smoothie, 72
Green Beans Amandine, 98
Grilled Eggplant Burgers, 127
Ground Lamb and
    Lentil Chili, 165
Guacamole, 207

H

Halibut and Veggie
    Packets, 136
Hamburger Stew, 160
Hamburger Stroganoff with
    Zucchini Noodles, 159
Herb-Crusted Lamb
    Chops, 166
Honeydew and Cilantro
    Ice Pops, 184

I

Inside-Out Cabbage Rolls, 158
Italian Vegetable Soup, 111

K

Kale, Oregano, and Pine
    Nut Pesto, 202

L

Lamb and Chickpea
    Stew, 168
Lamb Meatballs with Lemon
    Yogurt Sauce, 164
Lemon Yogurt Sauce, 199
Lentil Tacos, 116

M

Maple-Ginger Oatmeal, 76
Maple-Glazed Salmon, 139
Mashed Potatoes, 101
Melon Granita, 183
Melon with Ginger Dipping
    Sauce, 182
Miso-Glazed Scallops, 133
Miso Soup with Tofu
    and Greens, 110
Mushroom and Herb
    Omelet, 88

O

Olive Tapenade, 95
One-Pot Chicken Stew, 147
Open-Faced Stuffed
    Burgers, 169
Oregano and Parsley
    Chimichurri, 205
Oven-Fried Chicken, 145

P

Papaya Vinaigrette, 196
Pasta with Walnut Pesto, 117
Patty Melt Soup, 156
Peanut and Carob Balls, 180
Peanut Butter and
    Banana Spread
    with Ginger, 181
Peanut Butter Cookies, 190
Pesto Grilled Cheese, 128
Pho with Beef and
    Zucchini Noodles, 155
Poultry Broth, 195
Puffy Omelet, 89

Q

Quick Chicken and Veggie
    Stir-Fry, 146
Quick Pasta Salad, 105
Quinoa Pilaf, 102

R

Raisin Cornmeal Pancakes, 78

Roasted Asparagus with
    Goat Cheese, 99
Roasted Honey-Ginger
    Carrots, 103
Roasted Lamb Chops with
    Chimichurri, 167

S

Salmon and Egg Scramble, 87
Salmon and Lentils, 140
Shepherd's Pie Muffins, 163
Simple Vegetable Broth, 108
Sirloin Steak Salad with
    Papaya Vinaigrette, 157
Soba Noodles with Peanut
    Butter Sauce, 121
Spiced Walnuts, 173
Spinach and Dill Dip, 92
Spinach Frittata, 86
Steamer Clams with
    Fennel, 135
Stir-Fry Sauce, 204
Sweet Melon Smoothie, 71
Sweet Potato and Corn
    Stew, 114
Sweet Potato French Fries, 96
Sweet Potato Hash, 81

T

Tartar Sauce, 197
Tilapia with Cantaloupe
    Salsa, 137
Toads in a Hole, 82

Tofu with Chimichurri, 126
Turkey and Egg Breakfast
    Sandwich, 83
Turkey and Spinach
    Rollatini, 151
Turkey Breakfast Sausage, 84
Turkey Meatballs, 149
Turkey Meatloaf Muffins, 150
Turkey-Wrapped Melon, 178

V

Vegetable and Tofu
    Fried Rice, 123
Vegetable Beef Soup, 154

W

Walnut-Basil Pesto, 201

Yogurt and Melon Ice Pops, 185
Yogurt Sour Cream, 208

Z

Zucchini and Carrot
    Frittata, 118
Zucchini and Salmon
    Canapés, 94
Zucchini Hummus, 93
Zucchini Ribbons with
    Parmesan Cream
    Sauce, 119

Index

A

Acidic foods, 8, 21
Acid rebound, 51
Acid reflux
  causes of, 6–8
  and connection to gut
    and diet, 11–16
  diet guidelines, 25–26
  lifestyle solutions for, 16–17
  symptoms, 8–9
  when to see a doctor, 9–11
Alkaline diets, 22
Aloe vera, 10, 44
  Green Aloe Vera
    Smoothie, 72
Anchovies
  Olive Tapenade, 95
Anti-inflammatory drinks, 27
Anti-inflammatory foods, 20
Appetizers. *See also* Snacks
  Olive Tapenade, 95
  Spinach and Dill Dip, 92
  Zucchini and Salmon
    Canapés, 94
  Zucchini Hummus, 93
Apples
  Apple Compote
    Smoothie, 75
Artichokes
  Artichoke Purée, 97
Artificial sweeteners, 25
Asparagus
  Roasted Asparagus with
    Goat Cheese, 99
Avocados
  Baked Avocado and
    Egg, 85
  Beef Tacos, 161
  Cooling Cucumber
    Soup, 109
  Guacamole, 207
  Lentil Tacos, 116

B

Baking soda, 51
Bananas
  Banana and Melon
    Salad, 188
  Banana-Flax Smoothie, 70
  Banana Ice Cream, 187
  Banana Pancakes, 80
  Banana Pudding, 191
  Brûléed Bananas, 186
  Fruit and Yogurt Parfait, 74
  Green Aloe Vera
    Smoothie, 72
  Peanut Butter and Banana
    Spread with Ginger, 181
Barrett's esophagus, 7
Basil
  Basil Dressing, 203
  Italian Vegetable Soup, 111
  Olive Tapenade, 95
  Open-Faced Stuffed
    Burgers, 169
  Pasta with Walnut Pesto, 117
  Quick Pasta Salad, 105
  Walnut-Basil Pesto, 201
Beans. *See also* Chickpeas;
  Green beans
  Italian Vegetable Soup, 111
Bean sprouts
  Pho with Beef and
    Zucchini Noodles, 155
Beef
  Beef Tacos, 161
  Flank Steak with
    Chimichurri, 162
  Hamburger Stew, 160
  Hamburger Stroganoff with
    Zucchini Noodles, 159
  Inside-Out Cabbage
    Rolls, 158
  Open-Faced Stuffed
    Burgers, 169
  Patty Melt Soup, 156
  Pho with Beef and
    Zucchini Noodles, 155
  Sirloin Steak Salad with
    Papaya Vinaigrette, 157
  Vegetable Beef Soup, 154
Beverages, 26–27
Bok choy
  Asian Veggie and Tofu
    Stir-Fry, 120
  Quick Chicken and
    Veggie Stir-Fry, 146
Bone broth, 10, 43
Bread
  Easy Tuna Melt, 138
  French Toast, 79
  Fried Egg Sandwich, 129
  Open-Faced Stuffed
    Burgers, 169
  Pesto Grilled Cheese, 128
  Toads in a Hole, 82
  Turkey and Egg Breakfast
    Sandwich, 83
Breakfasts. *See also*
  Smoothies
  Baked Avocado and Egg, 85
  Banana Pancakes, 80
  Chia Breakfast Pudding
    with Cantaloupe, 73

Breakfasts (*Continued*)
  Corn Porridge with Maple
    and Raisins, 77
  French Toast, 79
  Fruit and Yogurt Parfait, 74
  Maple-Ginger Oatmeal, 76
  Mushroom and Herb
    Omelet, 88
  Puffy Omelet, 89
  Raisin Cornmeal
    Pancakes, 78
  Salmon and Egg
    Scramble, 87
  Spinach Frittata, 86
  Sweet Potato Hash, 81
  Toads in a Hole, 82
  Turkey and Egg Breakfast
    Sandwich, 83
  Turkey Breakfast
    Sausage, 84
Broccoli
  Broccoli and Cheese
    Baked Potato, 115
  Cream of Broccoli Soup, 113
  Vegetable and Tofu
    Fried Rice, 123

C

Cabbage
  Inside-Out Cabbage
    Rolls, 158
Cantaloupe
  Banana and Melon
    Salad, 188
  Cantaloupe Salsa, 206
  Chia Breakfast Pudding
    with Cantaloupe, 73
  Melon Granita, 183
  Melon with Ginger
    Dipping Sauce, 182
  Sweet Melon Smoothie, 71
Carbohydrates, 13–14. *See
    also* FODMAPs

Carbonated beverages, 27
Carrots
  Asian Veggie and Tofu
    Stir-Fry, 120
  Beef Broth, 194
  Brown Rice and Tofu
    with Kale, 125
  Carrots with Herbed
    Yogurt Dip, 177
  Chicken Noodle Soup, 143
  Chopped Kale Salad, 104
  Fisherman's Stew, 142
  Grated Carrot and
    Raisin Salad, 179
  Hamburger Stew, 160
  Italian Vegetable
    Soup, 111
  Poultry Broth, 195
  Quick Chicken and
    Veggie Stir-Fry, 146
  Quinoa Pilaf, 102
  Roasted Honey-Ginger
    Carrots, 103
  Salmon and Lentils, 140
  Shepherd's Pie Muffins, 163
  Simple Vegetable Broth, 108
  Simple Vegetable and
    Tofu Fried Rice, 123
  Vegetable Beef Soup, 154
  Zucchini and Carrot
    Frittata, 118
Celery
  Chicken Noodle Soup, 143
  Poultry Broth, 195
  Simple Vegetable Broth, 108
Cheese
  Beef Tacos, 161
  Broccoli and Cheese
    Baked Potato, 115
  Butternut Risotto, 124
  Easy Tuna Melt, 138
  Fish Tacos with
    Guacamole, 141

Open-Faced Stuffed
    Burgers, 169
  Pasta with Walnut Pesto, 117
  Patty Melt Soup, 156
  Pesto Grilled Cheese, 128
  Roasted Asparagus with
    Goat Cheese, 99
  Shepherd's Pie Muffins, 163
  Turkey and Spinach
    Rollatini, 151
  Walnut-Basil Pesto, 201
  Zucchini Ribbons
    with Parmesan
    Cream Sauce, 119
Chia seeds
  Chia Breakfast Pudding
    with Cantaloupe, 73
Chicken
  Baked Chicken
    Tenders, 144
  Chicken Noodle Soup, 143
  One-Pot Chicken Stew, 147
  Oven-Fried Chicken, 145
  Poultry Broth, 195
  Quick Chicken and
    Veggie Stir-Fry, 146
Chickpeas
  Lamb and Chickpea
    Stew, 168
  Quick Pasta Salad, 105
Cilantro
  Brown Rice and Peanut
    Lettuce Wraps, 122
  Cantaloupe Salsa, 206
  Cooling Cucumber
    Soup, 109
  Fish Tacos with
    Guacamole, 141
  Flank Steak with
    Chimichurri, 162
  Ground Lamb and
    Lentil Chili, 165
  Guacamole, 207

Cilantro (*Continued*)
    Honeydew and Cilantro
      Ice Pops, 184
    Lentil Tacos, 116
    Pho with Beef and
      Zucchini Noodles, 155
    Quick Chicken and
      Veggie Stir-Fry, 146
    Soba Noodles with
      Peanut Butter Sauce, 121
    Sweet Potato and
      Corn Stew, 114
    Turkey Meatballs, 149
Coconut milk
    Creamy Pumpkin Soup, 112
    Soba Noodles with Peanut
      Butter Sauce, 121
Cooking tips, 59
Corn
    Hamburger Stew, 160
    Sweet Potato and
      Corn Stew, 114
Cornmeal
    Corn Porridge with
      Maple and Raisins, 77
    Raisin Cornmeal
      Pancakes, 78
Corn tortillas
    Beef Tacos, 161
    Fish Tacos with
      Guacamole, 141
    Lentil Tacos, 116
Cravings, 58–59
Cucumbers
    Cooling Cucumber
      Soup, 109
    Cucumber Rounds with
      Shrimp Salad, 175

D
Digestion
    overview, 4–5
    slow, and low stomach
      acid, 12–13

Digestive enzymes, 44
Dill
    Carrots with Herbed
      Yogurt Dip, 177
    Chopped Kale Salad, 104
    Crab Cakes with
      Tartar Sauce, 132
    Deviled Eggs, 172
    Salmon and Lentils, 140
    Spinach and Dill Dip, 92
    Tartar Sauce, 197
    Zucchini Hummus, 93
Dips and spreads
    Olive Tapenade, 95
    Peanut Butter and
      Banana Spread
      with Ginger, 181
    Spinach and Dill Dip, 92
    Zucchini Hummus, 93

E
Edamame
    Quick Chicken and
      Veggie Stir-Fry, 146
Eggplants
    Grilled Eggplant
      Burgers, 127
Eggs
    Almond Meringue
      Cookies, 189
    Baked Avocado and
      Egg, 85
    Deviled Eggs, 172
    Fried Egg Sandwich, 129
    Mushroom and Herb
      Omelet, 88
    Peanut Butter Cookies, 190
    Puffy Omelet, 89
    Salmon and Egg
      Scramble, 87
    Spinach Frittata, 86
    Toads in a Hole, 82
    Turkey and Egg Breakfast
      Sandwich, 83

    Zucchini and Carrot
      Frittata, 118
Equipment, 60

F
Fennel
    Beef Broth, 194
    Brown Rice and Tofu
      with Kale, 125
    Fisherman's Stew, 142
    One-Pot Chicken Stew, 147
    Simple Vegetable Broth, 108
    Steamer Clams with
      Fennel, 135
    Vegetable Beef Soup, 154
Fermentation,
    excessive, 13–14, 37
Fermented foods, 44
Fiber, 20–21
Fish
    Easy Tuna Melt, 138
    Fisherman's Stew, 142
    Fish Tacos with
      Guacamole, 141
    Halibut and Veggie
      Packets, 136
    Maple-Glazed Salmon, 139
    Olive Tapenade, 95
    Salmon and Egg
      Scramble, 87
    Salmon and Lentils, 140
    Tilapia with Cantaloupe
      Salsa, 137
    Zucchini and Salmon
      Canapés, 94
5-Ingredient recipes, 65
    Almond Meringue
      Cookies, 189
    Apple Compote
      Smoothie, 75
    Artichoke Purée, 97
    Baked Avocado
      and Egg, 85
    Baked Potato Chips, 176

5-Ingredient recipes
(*Continued*)
Banana and Melon
Salad, 188
Banana-Flax Smoothie, 70
Banana Ice Cream, 187
Banana Pancakes, 80
Banana Pudding, 191
Beef Broth, 194
Breaded Crispy Shrimp, 134
Broccoli and Cheese
Baked Potato, 115
Brûléed Bananas, 186
Burger Sauce, 198
Cantaloupe Salsa, 206
Chia Breakfast Pudding
with Cantaloupe, 73
Cinnamon-Sugar
Popcorn, 174
Corn Porridge with Maple
and Raisins, 77
Creamed Spinach, 100
Creamy Herbed
Dressing, 200
Cucumber Rounds with
Shrimp Salad, 175
Deviled Eggs, 172
Easy Tuna Melt, 138
Easy Turkey Burgers, 148
Fried Egg Sandwich, 129
Fruit and Yogurt
Parfait, 74
Grated Carrot and
Raisin Salad, 179
Green Aloe Vera
Smoothie, 72
Green Beans Amandine, 98
Grilled Eggplant
Burgers, 127
Guacamole, 207
Honeydew and Cilantro
Ice Pops, 184
Kale, Oregano, and Pine
Nut Pesto, 202

Lamb Meatballs with
Lemon Yogurt
Sauce, 164
Lemon Yogurt Sauce, 199
Maple-Ginger Oatmeal, 76
Maple-Glazed Salmon, 139
Mashed Potatoes, 101
Melon Granita, 183
Melon with Ginger
Dipping Sauce, 182
Miso-Glazed Scallops, 133
Miso Soup with Tofu
and Greens, 110
Mushroom and Herb
Omelet, 88
Olive Tapenade, 95
Oregano and Parsley
Chimichurri, 205
Oven-Fried Chicken, 145
Papaya Vinaigrette, 196
Pasta with Walnut Pesto, 117
Peanut and Carob Balls, 180
Peanut Butter and Banana
Spread with Ginger, 181
Peanut Butter Cookies, 190
Pesto Grilled Cheese, 128
Poultry Broth, 195
Puffy Omelet, 89
Roasted Asparagus with
Goat Cheese, 99
Roasted Honey-Ginger
Carrots, 103
Roasted Lamb Chops
with Chimichurri, 167
Salmon and Egg
Scramble, 87
Simple Vegetable Broth, 108
Sirloin Steak Salad
with Papaya
Vinaigrette, 157
Spiced Walnuts, 173
Spinach and Dill Dip, 92
Spinach Frittata, 86
Stir-Fry Sauce, 204

Sweet Melon Smoothie, 71
Sweet Potato French
Fries, 96
Sweet Potato Hash, 81
Tartar Sauce, 197
Tilapia with Cantaloupe
Salsa, 137
Toads in a Hole, 82
Tofu with Chimichurri, 126
Turkey and Egg Breakfast
Sandwich, 83
Turkey and Spinach
Rollatini, 151
Turkey Breakfast
Sausage, 84
Turkey Meatloaf
Muffins, 150
Turkey-Wrapped
Melon, 178
Walnut-Basil Pesto, 201
Yogurt and Melon
Ice Pops, 185
Yogurt Sour Cream, 208
Zucchini and Carrot
Frittata, 118
Zucchini and Salmon
Canapés, 94
Zucchini Hummus, 93
Zucchini Ribbons
with Parmesan
Cream Sauce, 119
Flare-ups, treating, 10
Flaxseed
Banana-Flax Smoothie, 70
FODMAPs, 13, 20, 23–24, 26
Food sensitivities, 15
Fructan, 23
Fructose, 23

G

Galactans, 23
Garlic
Garlic Oil, 209
Gastroenterologists, 9–11

GERD, 7, 8, 20–21. *See also*
    Acid reflux
Ginger, 10, 43, 59
    Asian Veggie and Tofu
        Stir-Fry, 120
    Brown Rice and Peanut
        Lettuce Wraps, 122
    Cooling Cucumber
        Soup, 109
    Maple-Ginger Oatmeal, 76
    Melon Granita, 183
    Melon with Ginger
        Dipping Sauce, 182
    Peanut Butter and Banana
        Spread with Ginger, 181
    Pho with Beef and
        Zucchini Noodles, 155
    Roasted Honey-Ginger
        Carrots, 103
    Soba Noodles with Peanut
        Butter Sauce, 121
    Stir-Fry Sauce, 204
    Turkey Meatballs, 149
    Vegetable and Tofu
        Fried Rice, 123
Green beans
    Green Beans Amandine, 98
    Italian Vegetable
        Soup, 111
    One-Pot Chicken
        Stew, 147
    Vegetable Beef Soup, 154
Gut flora, 5, 13–14, 21

H

Hamburger buns
    Easy Turkey Burgers, 148
    Grilled Eggplant
        Burgers, 127
HEAL plan, 26, 37–49
Heartburn
    causes of, 6–8
    flare-up remedies, 10
    symptoms, 8

Helicobacter pylori
    (H. pylori), 4, 12
Honey
    Chia Breakfast Pudding
        with Cantaloupe, 73
    Roasted Honey-Ginger
        Carrots, 103
Honeydew melon
    Honeydew and Cilantro
        Ice Pops, 184
    Melon Granita, 183
    Melon with Ginger
        Dipping Sauce, 182
    Turkey-Wrapped
        Melon, 178
    Yogurt and Melon
        Ice Pops, 185
Hydrochloric acid
    (HCl), 4–5, 12–13

I

Inflammation, 16
Intra-abdominal pressure
    (IAP), 7–8, 14

K

Kale
    Brown Rice and Tofu
        with Kale, 125
    Chopped Kale Salad, 104
    Cream of Broccoli
        Soup, 113
    Kale, Oregano, and Pine
        Nut Pesto, 202

L

Lactose, 23
Lamb
    Ground Lamb and
        Lentil Chili, 165
    Herb-Crusted Lamb
        Chops, 166
    Lamb and Chickpea
        Stew, 168

    Lamb Meatballs with
        Lemon Yogurt Sauce, 164
    Roasted Lamb Chops
        with Chimichurri, 167
    Shepherd's Pie Muffins, 163
    Simple Vegetable Broth, 108
Laryngopharyngeal reflux
    (LPR), 7, 8–9, 20–21.
        See also Acid reflux
Leeks
    Asian Veggie and Tofu
        Stir-Fry, 120
    Beef Tacos, 161
    Brown Rice and Peanut
        Lettuce Wraps, 122
    Brown Rice and
        Tofu with Kale, 125
    Chicken Noodle Soup, 143
    Cream of Broccoli Soup, 113
    Creamy Pumpkin Soup, 112
    Fisherman's Stew, 142
    Ground Lamb and
        Lentil Chili, 165
    Hamburger Stew, 160
    Hamburger Stroganoff with
        Zucchini Noodles, 159
    Inside-Out Cabbage
        Rolls, 158
    Italian Vegetable Soup, 111
    Lamb and Chickpea
        Stew, 168
    Lentil Tacos, 116
    Miso Soup with Tofu
        and Greens, 110
    One-Pot Chicken Stew, 147
    Patty Melt Soup, 156
    Poultry Broth, 195
    Quick Chicken and
        Veggie Stir-Fry, 146
    Shepherd's Pie Muffins, 163
    Steamer Clams with
        Fennel, 135
    Sweet Potato and
        Corn Stew, 114

Leeks (*Continued*)
    Vegetable and Tofu
        Fried Rice, 123
    Vegetable Beef Soup, 154
Lemon zest
    Carrots with Herbed
        Yogurt Dip, 177
    Crab Cakes with
        Tartar Sauce, 132
    Creamy Herbed
        Dressing, 200
    Green Beans Amandine, 98
    Halibut and Veggie
        Packets, 136
    Lemon Yogurt Sauce, 199
    Olive Tapenade, 95
    Oregano and Parsley
        Chimichurri, 205
    Papaya Vinaigrette, 196
    Pasta with Walnut
        Pesto, 117
    Roasted Asparagus with
        Goat Cheese, 99
    Spinach and Dill Dip, 92
    Steamer Clams with
        Fennel, 135
    Tartar Sauce, 197
    Turkey and Spinach
        Rollatini, 151
    Walnut-Basil Pesto, 201
    Zucchini Hummus, 93
Lentils
    Ground Lamb and
        Lentil Chili, 165
    Lentil Tacos, 116
    Salmon and Lentils, 140
Lettuce
    Brown Rice and Peanut
        Lettuce Wraps, 122
    Sirloin Steak Salad with
        Papaya Vinaigrette, 157
Lime zest
    Cantaloupe Salsa, 206

Cooling Cucumber
    Soup, 109
Fish Tacos with
    Guacamole, 141
Flank Steak with
    Chimichurri, 162
Ground Lamb and
    Lentil Chili, 165
Guacamole, 207
Honeydew and Cilantro
    Ice Pops, 184
Pho with Beef and
    Zucchini Noodles, 155
Sweet Potato and
    Corn Stew, 114
Yogurt Sour Cream, 208
Lower esophageal sphincter
    (LES), 4, 7, 14
LPR. *See* Laryngopharyngeal
    reflux (LPR)

M

Maple syrup
    Banana and Melon
        Salad, 188
    Banana Ice Cream, 187
    Corn Porridge with Maple
        and Raisins, 77
    Fruit and Yogurt Parfait, 74
    Grated Carrot and
        Raisin Salad, 179
    Maple-Ginger Oatmeal, 76
    Maple-Glazed Salmon, 139
    Melon Granita, 183
    Melon with Ginger
        Dipping Sauce, 182
    Miso-Glazed Scallops, 133
    Peanut Butter and
        Banana Spread
        with Ginger, 181
    Raisin Cornmeal
        Pancakes, 78
    Turkey-Wrapped Melon, 178

Yogurt and Melon
    Ice Pops, 185
Meal planning
    diet guidelines, 25–26
    HEAL plan, 37–49
    REINTRODUCE plan, 50–58
    STOP plan, 31–36
    tips, 30
Medications, 7, 12, 14
Meditation, 17
Milk, lactose-free
    Apple Compote
        Smoothie, 75
    Artichoke Purée, 97
    Banana-Flax Smoothie, 70
    Banana Pudding, 191
    Basil Dressing, 203
    Chia Breakfast
        Pudding with
        Cantaloupe, 73
    Creamed Spinach, 100
    Cream of Broccoli
        Soup, 113
    French Toast, 79
    Hamburger Stroganoff
        with Zucchini
        Noodles, 159
    Mashed Potatoes, 101
    Open-Faced Stuffed
        Burgers, 169
    Raisin Cornmeal
        Pancakes, 78
    Sweet Melon Smoothie, 71
    Turkey Meatballs, 149
    Zucchini Ribbons
        with Parmesan
        Cream Sauce, 119
Mushrooms
    Hamburger Stroganoff
        with Zucchini
        Noodles, 159
    Mushroom and Herb
        Omelet, 88

N

Nuts
Fruit and Yogurt Parfait, 74
Green Beans Amandine, 98
Kale, Oregano, and Pine
Nut Pesto, 202
Pasta with Walnut Pesto, 117
Quinoa Pilaf, 102
Spiced Walnuts, 173
Walnut-Basil Pesto, 201

O

Oats
Maple-Ginger Oatmeal, 76
Obesity, 14–16
Oils and fats, 35
Olives
Olive Tapenade, 95
Quick Pasta Salad, 105
Omega-3 fatty acids, 44
One-Pan recipes, 65
Asian Veggie and Tofu
Stir-Fry, 120
Baked Avocado and Egg, 85
Banana and Melon
Salad, 188
Banana-Flax Smoothie, 70
Banana Ice Cream, 187
Basil Dressing, 203
Broccoli and Cheese
Baked Potato, 115
Brown Rice and Peanut
Lettuce Wraps, 122
Brown Rice and Tofu
with Kale, 125
Brûléed Bananas, 186
Burger Sauce, 198
Cantaloupe Salsa, 206
Carrots with Herbed
Yogurt Dip, 177
Chia Breakfast Pudding
with Cantaloupe, 73
Chicken Noodle Soup, 143

Creamy Herbed
Dressing, 200
Cucumber Rounds with
Shrimp Salad, 175
Fried Egg Sandwich, 129
Grated Carrot and
Raisin Salad, 179
Green Aloe Vera
Smoothie, 72
Ground Lamb and
Lentil Chili, 165
Guacamole, 207
Halibut and Veggie
Packets, 136
Hamburger Stew, 160
Inside-Out Cabbage
Rolls, 158
Italian Vegetable Soup, 111
Kale, Oregano, and Pine
Nut Pesto, 202
Lemon Yogurt Sauce, 199
Lentil Tacos, 116
Maple-Ginger Oatmeal, 76
Mashed Potatoes, 101
Melon Granita, 183
Melon with Ginger
Dipping Sauce, 182
Mushroom and Herb
Omelet, 88
Olive Tapenade, 95
Oregano and Parsley
Chimichurri, 205
Papaya Vinaigrette, 196
Patty Melt Soup, 156
Peanut and Carob Balls, 180
Peanut Butter and Banana
Spread with Ginger, 181
Pesto Grilled Cheese, 128
Pho with Beef and
Zucchini Noodles, 155
Poultry Broth, 195
Quick Chicken and
Veggie Stir-Fry, 146

Quick Pasta Salad, 105
Quinoa Pilaf, 102
Roasted Asparagus with
Goat Cheese, 99
Salmon and Egg
Scramble, 87
Simple Vegetable Broth, 108
Soba Noodles with Peanut
Butter Sauce, 121
Spiced Walnuts, 173
Steamer Clams with
Fennel, 135
Stir-Fry Sauce, 204
Sweet Melon Smoothie, 71
Sweet Potato Hash, 81
Tartar Sauce, 197
Tilapia with Cantaloupe
Salsa, 137
Turkey and Egg Breakfast
Sandwich, 83
Turkey and Spinach
Rollatini, 151
Turkey-Wrapped
Melon, 178
Vegetable Beef Soup, 154
Walnut-Basil Pesto, 201
Yogurt Sour Cream, 208
Zucchini and Salmon
Canapés, 94
Zucchini Hummus, 93
One-Pot recipes, 65
Orange zest
Almond Meringue
Cookies, 189
Asian Veggie and Tofu
Stir-Fry, 120
Banana and Melon
Salad, 188
Basil Dressing, 203
Brown Rice and Tofu
with Kale, 125
Chopped Kale
Salad, 104

Orange zest (*Continued*)
  Corn Porridge with Maple
    and Raisins, 77
  Cucumber Rounds with
    Shrimp Salad, 175
  French Toast, 79
  Kale, Oregano, and Pine
    Nut Pesto, 202
  Lamb and Chickpea
    Stew, 168
  Maple-Glazed Salmon, 139
  Turkey-Wrapped Melon, 178
  Zucchini and Salmon
    Canapés, 94
Oregano
  Herb-Crusted Lamb
    Chops, 166
  Kale, Oregano, and Pine
    Nut Pesto, 202
  Oregano and Parsley
    Chimichurri, 205

P

Pantry staples, 61–62
Papaya, 44
  Papaya Vinaigrette, 196
Parsley
  Carrots with Herbed
    Yogurt Dip, 177
  Creamy Herbed
    Dressing, 200
  Flank Steak with
    Chimichurri, 162
  Green Aloe Vera
    Smoothie, 72
  Herb-Crusted Lamb
    Chops, 166
  Oregano and Parsley
    Chimichurri, 205
  Quinoa Pilaf, 102
  Salmon and Lentils, 140
Parsnips
  Salmon and Lentils, 140

Pasta
  Chicken Noodle Soup, 143
  Pasta with Walnut Pesto, 117
  Quick Pasta Salad, 105
Peanut butter
  Brown Rice and Peanut
    Lettuce Wraps, 122
  Peanut and Carob Balls, 180
  Peanut Butter and
    Banana Spread
    with Ginger, 181
  Peanut Butter Cookies, 190
  Soba Noodles with Peanut
    Butter Sauce, 121
Peas
  Shepherd's Pie Muffins, 163
Pepsin, 4, 7–8, 21, 35–36
pH, 21, 22
  FDA food lists, 211–214
Pineapple, 44
Polyols, 23
Popcorn
  Cinnamon-Sugar
    Popcorn, 174
Potatoes. *See also* Sweet
    potatoes
  Baked Potato Chips, 176
  Broccoli and Cheese
    Baked Potato, 115
  Fisherman's Stew, 142
  Hamburger Stew, 160
  Mashed Potatoes, 101
  One-Pot Chicken Stew, 147
Prebiotics, 24
Probiotics, 43
Proton pump inhibitors
    (PPIs), 7, 14
Pumpkin
  Creamy Pumpkin Soup, 112

Q

Quinoa
  Quinoa Pilaf, 102

R

Radishes
  Chopped Kale Salad, 104
Raisins
  Corn Porridge with Maple
    and Raisins, 77
  Grated Carrot and
    Raisin Salad, 179
  Quinoa Pilaf, 102
  Raisin Cornmeal
    Pancakes, 78
Recipe labels, 64–65
Reflux. *See also* Acid reflux
  causes of, 6–8
  symptoms, 8
Reflux Symptom Index
    (RSI), 8–9
REINTRODUCE
    plan, 26, 50–58
Rice
  Brown Rice and Peanut
    Lettuce Wraps, 122
  Brown Rice and Tofu
    with Kale, 125
  Butternut Risotto, 124
  Inside-Out Cabbage
    Rolls, 158
  Vegetable and Tofu
    Fried Rice, 123
Rosemary
  Beef Broth, 194
  Creamy Herbed
    Dressing, 200
  Herb-Crusted Lamb
    Chops, 166

S

Salads
  Banana and Melon
    Salad, 188
  Chopped Kale Salad, 104
  Cucumber Rounds
    with Shrimp Salad, 175

Salads (*Continued*)
Grated Carrot and
Raisin Salad, 179
Quick Pasta Salad, 105
Sirloin Steak Salad with
Papaya Vinaigrette, 157
Salmon
Fisherman's Stew, 142
Maple-Glazed Salmon, 139
Salmon and Egg
Scramble, 87
Salmon and Lentils, 140
Zucchini and Salmon
Canapés, 94
Sandwiches and wraps
Beef Tacos, 161
Brown Rice and Peanut
Lettuce Wraps, 122
Easy Tuna Melt, 138
Easy Turkey Burgers, 148
Fish Tacos with
Guacamole, 141
Fried Egg Sandwich, 129
Grilled Eggplant
Burgers, 127
Lentil Tacos, 116
Open-Faced Stuffed
Burgers, 169
Pesto Grilled
Cheese, 128
Turkey and Egg Breakfast
Sandwich, 83
Sauces and condiments
Basil Dressing, 203
Beef Broth, 194
Burger Sauce, 198
Cantaloupe Salsa, 206
Creamy Herbed
Dressing, 200
Garlic Oil, 209
Guacamole, 207
Kale, Oregano, and Pine
Nut Pesto, 202

Lemon Yogurt Sauce, 199
Oregano and Parsley
Chimichurri, 205
Papaya Vinaigrette, 196
Poultry Broth, 195
Simple Vegetable Broth, 108
Stir-Fry Sauce, 204
Tartar Sauce, 197
Walnut-Basil Pesto, 201
Yogurt Sour Cream, 208
Seafood. *See also* Fish
Breaded Crispy
Shrimp, 134
Crab Cakes with
Tartar Sauce, 132
Cucumber Rounds with
Shrimp Salad, 175
Miso-Glazed Scallops, 133
Steamer Clams with
Fennel, 135
Shrimp
Breaded Crispy Shrimp, 134
Crab Cakes with
Tartar Sauce, 132
Cucumber Rounds with
Shrimp Salad, 175
Sides
Artichoke Purée, 97
Creamed Spinach, 100
Green Beans Amandine, 98
Mashed Potatoes, 101
Quinoa Pilaf, 102
Roasted Asparagus with
Goat Cheese, 99
Roasted Honey-Ginger
Carrots, 103
Sweet Potato French Fries, 96
Silent acid reflux. *See*
Laryngopharyngeal
reflux (LPR)
Sleep apnea, 17
Small intestinal bacterial
overgrowth (SIBO), 13–14

Smoothies
Apple Compote
Smoothie, 75
Banana-Flax Smoothie, 70
Green Aloe Vera
Smoothie, 72
Sweet Melon Smoothie, 71
Snacks. *See also* Appetizers
Baked Potato Chips, 176
Banana and Melon
Salad, 188
Carrots with Herbed
Yogurt Dip, 177
Cinnamon-Sugar
Popcorn, 174
Deviled Eggs, 172
Melon with Ginger
Dipping Sauce, 182
Peanut and Carob Balls, 180
Peanut Butter and Banana
Spread with Ginger, 181
Spiced Walnuts, 173
Turkey-Wrapped
Melon, 178
Soba noodles
Soba Noodles with Peanut
Butter Sauce, 121
Sodium bicarbonate, 51
Soups and stews
Chicken Noodle Soup, 143
Cooling Cucumber
Soup, 109
Cream of Broccoli Soup, 113
Creamy Pumpkin Soup, 112
Fisherman's Stew, 142
Ground Lamb and
Lentil Chili, 165
Hamburger Stew, 160
Italian Vegetable Soup, 111
Miso Soup with Tofu
and Greens, 110
One-Pot Chicken Stew, 147
Patty Melt Soup, 156

Soups and stews (*Continued*)
  Pho with Beef and
    Zucchini Noodles, 155
  Simple Vegetable Broth, 108
  Sweet Potato and
    Corn Stew, 114
  Vegetable Beef Soup, 154
Spinach
  Cooling Cucumber
    Soup, 109
  Creamed Spinach, 100
  Green Aloe Vera
    Smoothie, 72
  Miso Soup with Tofu
    and Greens, 110
  Quick Pasta Salad, 105
  Spinach and Dill Dip, 92
  Spinach Frittata, 86
  Sweet Potato and
    Corn Stew, 114
  Turkey and Spinach
    Rollatini, 151
Squash. *See also* Zucchini
  Butternut Risotto, 124
Stomach acid, 4–5, 12–13
STOP plan, 26, 31–36
Stress, 16, 17
Substitutions, 62–63
Sweet potatoes
  Sweet Potato and
    Corn Stew, 114
  Sweet Potato French
    Fries, 96
  Sweet Potato
    Hash, 81
Sweets
  Almond Meringue
    Cookies, 189
  Banana and Melon
    Salad, 188
  Banana Ice Cream, 187
  Banana Pudding, 191
  Brûléed Bananas, 186

Honeydew and Cilantro
  Ice Pops, 184
Melon Granita, 183
Melon with Ginger
  Dipping Sauce, 182
Peanut and Carob Balls, 180
Peanut Butter and Banana
  Spread with Ginger, 181
Peanut Butter Cookies, 190
Yogurt and Melon
  Ice Pops, 185

T

Tarragon
  Cucumber Rounds with
    Shrimp Salad, 175
  Turkey-Wrapped
    Melon, 178
  Zucchini and Salmon
    Canapés, 94
30-Minute recipes, 65
  Artichoke Purée, 97
  Asian Veggie and Tofu
    Stir-Fry, 120
  Baked Avocado and Egg, 85
  Baked Chicken Tenders, 144
  Baked Potato Chips, 176
  Banana and Melon
    Salad, 188
  Banana-Flax Smoothie, 70
  Banana Ice Cream, 187
  Banana Pancakes, 80
  Basil Dressing, 203
  Beef Tacos, 161
  Breaded Crispy Shrimp, 134
  Brown Rice and Peanut
    Lettuce Wraps, 122
  Brown Rice and Tofu
    with Kale, 125
  Brûléed Bananas, 186
  Burger Sauce, 198
  Butternut Risotto, 124
  Cantaloupe Salsa, 206

Carrots with Herbed
  Yogurt Dip, 177
Chicken Noodle Soup, 143
Chopped Kale Salad, 104
Cinnamon-Sugar
  Popcorn, 174
Corn Porridge with Maple
  and Raisins, 77
Crab Cakes with
  Tartar Sauce, 132
Creamed Spinach, 100
Cream of Broccoli Soup, 113
Creamy Herbed
  Dressing, 200
Creamy Pumpkin Soup, 112
Cucumber Rounds with
  Shrimp Salad, 175
Deviled Eggs, 172
Easy Tuna Melt, 138
Easy Turkey Burgers, 148
Fisherman's Stew, 142
Fish Tacos with
  Guacamole, 141
Flank Steak with
  Chimichurri, 162
French Toast, 79
Fried Egg Sandwich, 129
Fruit and Yogurt Parfait, 74
Grated Carrot and
  Raisin Salad, 179
Green Aloe Vera
  Smoothie, 72
Green Beans Amandine, 98
Grilled Eggplant
  Burgers, 127
Ground Lamb and
  Lentil Chili, 165
Guacamole, 207
Halibut and Veggie
  Packets, 136
Hamburger Stew, 160
Hamburger Stroganoff with
  Zucchini Noodles, 159

30-Minute recipes (*Continued*)
  Herb-Crusted Lamb
    Chops, 166
  Inside-Out Cabbage
    Rolls, 158
  Italian Vegetable Soup, 111
  Kale, Oregano, and Pine
    Nut Pesto, 202
  Lamb and Chickpea
    Stew, 168
  Lamb Meatballs with
    Lemon Yogurt Sauce, 164
  Lemon Yogurt Sauce, 199
  Lentil Tacos, 116
  Maple-Ginger Oatmeal, 76
  Maple-Glazed Salmon, 139
  Mashed Potatoes, 101
  Melon Granita, 183
  Melon with Ginger
    Dipping Sauce, 182
  Miso-Glazed Scallops, 133
  Miso Soup with Tofu
    and Greens, 110
  Mushroom and Herb
    Omelet, 88
  Olive Tapenade, 95
  One-Pot Chicken Stew, 147
  Oregano and Parsley
    Chimichurri, 205
  Papaya Vinaigrette, 196
  Pasta with Walnut Pesto, 117
  Patty Melt Soup, 156
  Peanut and Carob Balls, 180
  Peanut Butter and Banana
    Spread with Ginger, 181
  Peanut Butter Cookies, 190
  Pesto Grilled Cheese, 128
  Pho with Beef and
    Zucchini Noodles, 155
  Puffy Omelet, 89
  Quick Chicken and
    Veggie Stir-Fry, 146
  Quick Pasta Salad, 105

Quinoa Pilaf, 102
Raisin Cornmeal
  Pancakes, 78
Roasted Asparagus with
  Goat Cheese, 99
Roasted Honey-Ginger
  Carrots, 103
Roasted Lamb Chops
  with Chimichurri, 167
Salmon and Egg
  Scramble, 87
Salmon and Lentils, 140
Shepherd's Pie Muffins, 163
Sirloin Steak Salad with
  Papaya Vinaigrette, 157
Soba Noodles with Peanut
  Butter Sauce, 121
Spiced Walnuts, 173
Spinach and Dill Dip, 92
Spinach Frittata, 86
Steamer Clams with
  Fennel, 135
Stir-Fry Sauce, 204
Sweet Melon Smoothie, 71
Sweet Potato and
  Corn Stew, 114
Sweet Potato French
  Fries, 96
Sweet Potato Hash, 81
Tartar Sauce, 197
Tilapia with Cantaloupe
  Salsa, 137
Toads in a Hole, 82
Tofu with Chimichurri, 126
Turkey and Egg Breakfast
  Sandwich, 83
Turkey Breakfast
  Sausage, 84
Turkey Meatballs, 149
Turkey-Wrapped Melon, 178
Vegetable and Tofu
  Fried Rice, 123
Vegetable Beef Soup, 154

Walnut-Basil Pesto, 201
Yogurt Sour Cream, 208
Zucchini and Carrot
  Frittata, 118
Zucchini and Salmon
  Canapés, 94
Zucchini Hummus, 93
Zucchini Ribbons
  with Parmesan
  Cream Sauce, 119
Thyme
  Beef Broth, 194
  Burger Sauce, 198
  Carrots with Herbed
    Yogurt Dip, 177
  Chopped Kale
    Salad, 104
  Creamy Herbed
    Dressing, 200
  Papaya Vinaigrette, 196
  Zucchini and Carrot
    Frittata, 118
Tofu
  Asian Veggie and Tofu
    Stir-Fry, 120
  Brown Rice and Peanut
    Lettuce Wraps, 122
  Miso Soup with Tofu
    and Greens, 110
  Tofu with Chimichurri,
    126
  Vegetable and Tofu
    Fried Rice, 123
Turkey
  Easy Turkey Burgers, 148
  Poultry Broth, 195
  Turkey and Egg Breakfast
    Sandwich, 83
  Turkey and Spinach
    Rollatini, 151
  Turkey Breakfast
    Sausage, 84
  Turkey Meatballs, 149

Turkey (*Continued*)
    Turkey Meatloaf
        Muffins, 150
    Turkey-Wrapped Melon, 178

W

Water, 26–27

Y

Yogurt, lactose-free, 43–44
    Basil Dressing, 203
    Burger Sauce, 198
    Carrots with Herbed
        Yogurt Dip, 177
    Chopped Kale Salad, 104
    Cooling Cucumber
        Soup, 109
    Crab Cakes with
        Tartar Sauce, 132
    Cream of Broccoli Soup, 113
    Creamy Herbed
        Dressing, 200

Cucumber Rounds with
    Shrimp Salad, 175
Deviled Eggs, 172
Easy Tuna Melt, 138
Fruit and Yogurt
    Parfait, 74
Grated Carrot and
    Raisin Salad, 179
Honeydew and
    Cilantro Ice Pops, 184
Lemon Yogurt Sauce, 199
Melon with Ginger
    Dipping Sauce, 182
Spinach and Dill
    Dip, 92
Sweet Melon Smoothie, 71
Sweet Potato and
    Corn Stew, 114
Tartar Sauce, 197
Yogurt and Melon
    Ice Pops, 185
Yogurt Sour Cream, 208

Zucchini and Salmon
    Canapés, 94

Z

Zucchini
    Halibut and Veggie
        Packets, 136
    Hamburger Stroganoff
        with Zucchini
        Noodles, 159
    Italian Vegetable
        Soup, 111
    Pho with Beef and
        Zucchini Noodles, 155
    Zucchini and Carrot
        Frittata, 118
    Zucchini and Salmon
        Canapés, 94
    Zucchini Hummus, 93
    Zucchini Ribbons
        with Parmesan
        Cream Sauce, 119

Acknowledgments

I would like to thank the people who helped me be where I am today: My family for their continued support, my colleagues for their encouragement and for sharing their knowledge and expertise, Karen Frazier for collaborating on the recipes, the editing team for making this book a reality, and my wonderful patients who trusted me with their care.

About the Author

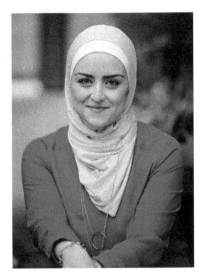

Nour Zibdeh, MS, RDN, CLT, is a registered dietitian and functional nutritionist, author, and speaker. She specializes in integrative nutrition therapies for digestive conditions, thyroid and hormone imbalances, autoimmune diseases, food sensitivities, migraines and headaches, chronic fatigue, chronic pain, and fibromyalgia. In her book, *The Detox Way*, Nour shares more than 100 real food, gluten- and dairy-free recipes for overall holistic health. Nour can be reached on her website at NourZibdeh.com, on Facebook at facebook.com/Nourition, or on YouTube at youtube.com/NourZibdeh.

Printed in the USA
CPSIA information can be obtained
at www.ICGtesting.com
CBHW081058120224
R14898500001B/R148985PG4145CBX00005B/7

9 781939 754790